Sadi

with best wishes

Michael Greenwood

# BRAVING THE VOID

*Pain is a fire which incinerates karma*
*And fuels evolutionary change*

— Lonny Jarrett

First edition.

Published by
PARADOX Publishers
1980 Cromwell Road
Victoria, BC V8P 1R5

If this book is not available through your bookstore, it may be ordered from the publisher. Send the cover price plus $4 for shipping.

Printed in Canada

ISBN 0-9695822-1-8

Editing, typesetting and page design, Susan Clark, A Use for Poets (Editing) Co., Vancouver.
Cover illustration by Miles Lowry.
Cover design by Jud Ridout, happydesigns, Victoria.

Canadian Cataloguing in Publication Data

Greenwood, Michael T. (Michael Tebay), 1949-
    Braving the void: journeys into healing

1st ed.
Includes index.
ISBN 0-9695822-1-8

    1. Healing.  2. Mind and body.  3. Mental healing.
I. Title.

## ABOUT THE AUTHOR

Dr. Michael Greenwood, M.B., B.Chir., C.C.F.P., C.A.F.C.I., F.R.S.A. was born in Singapore and raised in Victoria, BC. His lifelong ambition was to become a physician and he trained at St. John's College, Cambridge and St. Mary's Hospital, London University, then interned at the Royal Jubilee Hospital in Victoria. Later, he worked for a year in rural Australia before returning to Victoria to practise Family Medicine.

Michael's own experience of chronic pain began with a motorcycle accident while he was a medical student. The pain, unresponsive to all that conventional medicine could offer, forced him to face the limits of his own medical training. His search for an answer led him on a fascinating journey to a new understanding of health and illness, stress and deep inner tensions, and how they affect our lives. Those insights were recorded in Michael's first book, *Paradox and Healing*, co-authored with Dr. Peter Nunn and published in 1992.

In 1993, Michael gave up his Family Practice after seventeen years to devote his time to patients with chronic illness, developing experiential techniques which which integrate body, mind and spirit. His practice now encompasses acupuncture, bodywork, Traditional Chinese Medicine, and Ayurveda, and he works as Medical Director of the Victoria Pain Clinic, where he guides patients in what is frequently their first encounter with complementary medicine.

Michael and his wife Cherie live in Victoria, BC with their two sons, Mischa and Richard.

# BRAVING *the* VOID

journeys into healing

———

Michael Greenwood

# CONTENTS

## ACKNOWLEDGEMENTS

I have been most fortunate to work with a group of remarkable people. Without their various talents and the atmosphere of trust and safety they provide our clients, I doubt whether many of the extraordinary healing journeys I have been privileged to witness could possibly have occurred. In that respect, I would like to acknowledge the following people: first and foremost my wife, Cherie, whose tireless support over the years has led me onward into this fascinating arena of healing; Jean and Ken White — founders of the Victoria Pain Clinic — who have provided me with the ideal environment to help people safely explore their deep emotional issues; and my colleagues at the clinic: Tracey Nigro, our office manager; Darwyn Rowland, who with consummate skill in Hellerwork lets his fingers do the talking; Karen Snyder, who teaches biofeedback and has a special gift of healing in her hands; and Fiona Walker, whose delectable massages are everyone's delight.

I would like to make particular and heartfelt acknowledgement of my colleague and friend, Mary Joan Zakovy. Mary Joan works closely with me doing integrated bodywork, and has played a central role in many of the stories in this book. Her varied skills, which include counselling, psychotherapy and hypnotherapy, and her familiarity with non-rational states of consciousness provide a near-perfect balance to the objective physician in me. To her I owe a huge debt of gratitude. At the very least, the presence of both masculine and feminine energies during bodywork provides an unusually safe crucible for journeying into the void. However, Mary Joan brings far more than that to our work. Her enlivening presence, dedication to freedom and remarkable intuitive ability have inspired many people to dig far deeper than they otherwise might have considered possible. Although she is only mentioned on occasion throughout the book, her active presence as part of the matrix of many of the stories may be assumed.

The other member of the team who deserves a special note is Linda Wyness, who lives in residence during the program, and who is without a doubt one of the most experienced chronic pain counsellors around. She has been with the clinic since its inception in 1981, when

Peter and Heather Nunn founded the Victoria Stress and Pain Centre. Linda's remarkable wisdom and tireless support of clients during their journey of healing is something which could never be replaced.

My thanks also to Miles Lowry who contributed his vision to the cover art, to Jud Ridout, who designed the cover, and to David Ferguson who helped brainstorm the title of the book. To other colleagues at the clinic both past and present: Willow, Bert Proulx, Lonny Fox, Helen Jarvis, Diane Woodruff, Donna Ray, and Diane Smith. To Susan Clark, who gently prompted me to explore my own biases while skilfully editing the manuscript, and to Michael Gregson, who helped bring the whole project to completion, by guiding me through the complexities of publishing.

## NOTE

Although the stories in *Braving the Void* are based on the experiences of actual people, the names and many specific details of each case have been altered to protect their identities.

*for my father*

# Introduction

When I was a twenty-two-year-old medical student at St. Mary's Hospital in London, I was involved in a motorcycle accident. It was pub closing time and I was cruising down a one-way street in Lewisham, a suburb of south London, when a car pulled out from the curb and did a U-turn right in front of me. I was on my way home from a wedding at which I had had somewhat too much to drink and recall taking minimal evasive action, proceeding as if in slow motion straight into the collision. My left leg went numb as the bumper struck somewhere in mid-shin and I flew over the hood of the car and landed on the other side of the street. As I settled into the road, I could hear the sound of my motorbike crunching into the pavement and the roar of the car as it sped off in the opposite direction, the wrong way up the one-way street.

I remember being aware of two powerful feelings immediately after the impact. Conscious that I had done very little to avoid the accident, I was overwhelmed by a sense that the experience had profound meaning. And just for a moment — as I was flying over the hood of the car and seemed to hang in that void-like space between life as I'd known it and possible annihilation — I felt suddenly and fully alive in a way I have never experienced since.

Many years later, I had the opportunity to explore the chronic pain that resulted from the accident. During deep tissue work, as the therapist probed the scar on my leg — pushing the edge of my pain as far as I could tolerate — I returned to that moment. Breathing deeply to enter rather than resist the pain, I gradually broke through to a different consciousness. I found myself riding my old motorbike down the highway again, the wind in my face and — as too often happened — the rain in my boots. I could even feel my right wrist twisting as I primed the throttle, enjoying my adventure. Then, after a few minutes, I found myself again in Lewisham late at night on that familiar one-way street, my own voice imitating the sound of the humming engine.

It was all surprisingly real and though my rational mind knew perfectly well I was lying quite safely in a comfortable office, out of nowhere a car appeared in front of me. I felt myself hit the bumper and fly over the hood of the car, heard the terrible crunch of my dear motorcycle on the pavement — and felt once again that extraordinary sense of my life's meaning, this time with the rich affirmation and understanding of hindsight.

Though I wonder how I could have known it at the time, it's perfectly clear to me now that no event could have been more meaningful in the context of my life, given that I now work wholly with the sort of chronic conditions with which the accident left me. That accident was a turning point in my life and began the journey which took the young student of conventional medicine I was then through twenty-odd years of allopathic and alternative practices to the writer of the somewhat unconventional book you now hold in your hands.

For it seems that though we instinctively flee pain, we need not. Like so many of my clients, I have come to understand that at their deepest level our symptoms are often thresholds to the discovery of ourselves, that however fearful, they are potentially nothing less than gifts to be embraced. Pain, it seems, asks only that we do not reject it but invite it to reveal its great secret. By embracing pain, we can discover who we really are and allow our pain to become the greatest boon our lives have to offer.

I hope the fascinating case histories I have the privilege to be familiar with and to share with readers of *Braving the Void* will illustrate the courageous and trusting exploration necessary to initiate true healing and will inspire confidence by their examples.

Though *Braving the Void* may be difficult for some readers to absorb or accept, if it inspires a just few to pursue the road of healing, it will have been worth the writing.

*Michael Greenwood*
*Victoria, British Columbia*

Part I

———

POWER

*and*

HEALING

## Chapter I

# BEYOND PARADOX

*Beyond paradox lies the void*
*Where no answers are needed*
*Because there are no questions*

*M*any years ago when I was visiting South Africa, a physician friend told me a remarkable story. The story was about a Zulu woman who had refused life-saving surgery after a violent sexual assault. It seems she had been badly injured internally and was haemorrhaging so severely that emergency surgery was her only chance of survival. The surgery would include the removal of her uterus. As the woman already had several children, my friend and his Western-trained colleagues assumed she would willingly sacrifice it to save her life and were astonished when the woman emphatically refused the operation, saying that the removal of her womb would be a fate worse than death itself.

But the story didn't end there. The perplexed doctors watched their patient's condition deteriorate until it was clear that her death was imminent then decided to perform the lifesaving surgery without her consent, no doubt telling themselves she didn't really understand the gravity of the situation. The operation was successful and the medical staff expected a full recovery. But to their amazement, the woman did not revive. She refused to eat, went inexorably downhill and soon died anyway despite the fact that there was nothing wrong with her from a medical point of view.

I wondered why anyone would prefer to die rather than live on without a particular organ. No one even had to know what had been removed, I reasoned, trying to make sense of an incomprehensible situation and realizing dimly that I must be missing the point. But my friend was wiser. He said he and his colleagues were constantly surprised in their daily encounters with clients that procedures which Western medicine considers quite ordinary could have unpredictable effects when the belief system of the patient was left out of consideration. Slowly but surely, he told me, they were being made to understand that they had to respect cultural values *as though they were an integral part* of the person they were treating: as though beliefs were no less vital than organs.

My friend's story and his conclusion made a big impression on me and over the years I have come to feel that it is not just a story about a misunderstanding between one particular South African culture and Western medicine but a lesson for all who hope to heal or to be healed. It seems clear that we cannot aspire to remedy bodily illness if we studiously ignore the mind and spirit, the beliefs and the assumptions which inform our patients' personal cultures. And yet Western medicine still carries on, by and large, as if our minds and spirits were not part of bodily health and of illness.

## SCIENCE — THE WESTERN WORLD'S CULTURAL BIAS

As a culture, of course, we in the West are as much influenced by our belief system as my friend's Zulu patient. In fact, behind many of our chronic illnesses lies a wall of unshakeable cultural superstitions — opinions and ideas shared and supported by our health practitioners — which may entrap us in illness precisely because we can't or won't question them. Unfortunately, this deference both to the "Aesculapian authority"[1]

---

1. Aesculapius (Asclepius), Greek god of healing, father of Hygieia (hence *hygiene*), is represented by two snakes twined around a caduceus, or staff. "Aesculapian authority" refers to the authority invested in physicians and the medical establishment.

of the medical profession and to the cultural assumptions that underwrite it makes virtually impossible any encounter with health-giving new perspectives. Bound to our society's scientific bias, for instance, we find ourselves continually searching for the elusive "cause" of chronic symptoms. Where there is an effect, there must be a cause, reason tells us; and even when we have thoroughly exhausted the possibilities, we seem incapable of reckoning with the unpalatable truth that there may be no cause — at least not of the sort we may be seeking.

More often than not, there is no particular answer to the question of "cause" because it is really the wrong question. Once we understand and accept that illness is a part of ourselves, there may be no way to separate its "cause" from the illness, nor the illness from us. In other words, when dis-ease is disease, and disease is dis-ease, we are chasing our tails to ask "Why?" Rather than search for cause, then, better questions might be "Who am I?", "Why do I hurt?", or "What are my symptoms trying to tell me?" After all, if we do not know who we are, we have little chance of knowing why we are sick.

It takes a brave soul to defy the Aesculapian authority and great technical knowledge of modern medicine and set out instead on a quest for understanding. But let us look at some of the assumptions on which this authority is based. Healing — once considered a human art or a divine gift — is now only one expression of our society's profound and nearly universal commitment to the values of modern science. It may seem surprising then that much of the medicine which is practised today is still based on beliefs which were long ago disproved by that same science!

One of those beliefs, of course, is Western science's foundation stone: objectivity. The naïve lust for ever more precise "knowledge" of the world around us which has characterized the modern era has allowed science to flatter and delude itself.

Like the earth, static in the middle of the pre-Copernican solar system, science has assumed itself to be the autonomous centre of all it surveyed. And with hardly a blush has decked this autonomy out in the godly attributes of disembodied objectivity and all-seeing omniscience.

Our belief in cause and effect alluded to above and our assumption of a mind/body split — an assumption so ingrained that even those who profess holism often *behave* as if the split in fact exists — complete the Westerner's standard set of biases. In my first book, *Paradox and Healing* (co-authored with Peter Nunn), I discussed the existence of two "realities": what I call the "Cartesian perspective" — the separation of consciousness and matter — and its "inferred opposite." And I imagined them facing each other across a void or chasm. On one side, I saw the mind/body split; on the other, the body-mind connected. On one side was objectivity; on the other, subjectivity. Across an unbridgeable darkness, I imagined the rational and the irrational, linear vs. non-linear thinking, separation vs. connection, intellect vs. feeling, doing vs. being, masculine vs. feminine, illness vs. wellness, life vs. death — all that science has insisted on setting up as natural antitheses, in other words — standing inert and static on either side of a kind of void. It was some time before I realized that the void was all there really was, that the division was a totally artificial construct of my own Cartesian bias!

The essential point in that first book was that there are at least two ways of perceiving the world in which we live, and that in the West most of us are conditioned by upbringing and education to champion the rational and linear way (along with all its presumed correlates, the masculine, the intellectual and the active) as the "right" way. In fact, we take the Cartesian world view not merely as a correct view but as "the case" and "self-evident," as if it were itself a part of the real world and not merely one way of looking at it.

Unfortunately, this view tends to see the world in terms of visible matter and mass: it sees objects as strictly separate from each other and acknowledges no underlying connection between them. The "subjective" mode, on the other hand, describes a connected, energetic world view in which the perceiver is understood as part of — rather than separate from and looking onto — an infinitely complex and minutely interdependent web of relations.

So, though the Zulu woman's beliefs might seem incredible to a Western doctor, she might well find equally incredible his belief system's insistence on treating any given body part as though it had no relation to the rest of the body, nor to the emotional or spiritual self, and its larger context, its society. On the contrary, her apparent intransigence might put us on notice to pay attention to our own limitations.

This is not to suggest we must abandon the scientific knowledge acquired so painstakingly over the past few centuries but rather that we might aspire to better understand what it means to be human before we jump to scientific conclusions. If medicine is to help us really heal, we need to do some inner work to balance the excessive scientific focus on the outer. Such an approach might not have altered the fate of the Zulu woman but it would have allowed her to meet her destiny with dignity.

BEYOND OPPOSING PERSPECTIVES — TOWARD HEALING

The integration of inner and outer means bringing together the objective Cartesian world view with its supposed opposite, the energetic subjective view. To do that, we must give our rational minds a rest, stop trying to explain everything and let ourselves go beyond the problem of opposition altogether. Only then can we ask meaningful questions as to why we are ill.

Beyond paradox — that is, beyond all the seeming contradictions we cannot resolve — we encounter the "void" and explore an awesome world without dimensions or known limits, a world which speaks to us as nothing else can. The void, which I will describe more fully in the next chapter, is really a state of consciousness in which we can experience reality without the usual imposition of pattern recognition, based on the memory of similar forms we have come across in the past. When we enter the void, we begin to see beyond our habitual points-of-view and glimpse the underlying mystery of which we are a part.

The void is probably the simplest and most freely available, yet least understood, therapeutic tool available to those who wish to explore it. Moreover, its use returns healing power to the place where it belongs — to ourselves. That it is not more commonly utilized as a tool for healing — in spite of its benefits — speaks to the enormous fear we all carry around of taking responsibility for our symptoms and our experiences. A sincere exploration of the void takes us into the terror of completely unknown territory and shakes the foundations of our very firmest convictions.

## THE DESCENT INTO CHAOS

In my work as a physician, I began with the conscious desire to "fix" the seemingly isolated physical problems with which I was presented by my patients. But over the years I have come to understand that this approach — while it may appear to function well enough in acute medicine — teaches neither patient nor practitioner anything about themselves and is therefore no response at all to chronic illness or chronic pain. On the contrary, I have repeatedly seen that lasting solutions to chronic problems invariably involve a profound transformation of mind and spirit. It is as if these engrossing riddles of irremediable pain and illness present themselves most importantly as *invitations to a greater understanding of ourselves* and only secondarily as physical phenomena.

This seems to be the philosophical explanation of the remarkable journeys of healing I have witnessed. Until a profound shift in an individual's understanding occurs — a shift often necessitating a descent into the chaos of unresolved traumas, an examination of emotional "baggage," and a confrontation with previously unexamined cultural assumptions — no real healing occurs.

Much of the material for this book has come from working directly with clients who have abandoned attention to superficial symptoms and fruitless searches for a specific "cause" and a "quick fix," and have instead actively engaged in exploring the symptoms they intensely fear, through the heightened attention of the void. They have chosen to turn and confront themselves, owning their dis-ease as *a part of* that self.

Such healing is not for the capricious or the timid. It requires sincerity, courage and sustained commitment; and its course is unpredictable. The context of such exploration is therefore all-important. None of the work or the therapeutic relationships described in the following pages can be properly understood without reference to the environment in which those experiences and relationships occurred.

THE PHYSICIAN-PATIENT RELATIONSHIP

The journey of deep healing is, as we've said, often both arduous and terrifying, involving confrontations with long-buried feelings of grief, anger and fear as well as with our sexuality and with memories suppressed as insupportable. Patently, the traditional clinical relationship, which revolves around short, scheduled, one-on-one appointments, is not conducive to such journeys, even given the best of practitioners and the most committed of clients. An individual who has to function in the outer world at the end of an hour-long appointment simply cannot afford to risk a descent into repressed trauma.

Add to that a loss of trust in the medical establishment, fears concerning confidentiality and the anger at the invalidation of their experiences which most chronic pain sufferers feel, and it becomes clear that the conventional therapeutic environment can by itself be enough to interfere with the body's natural healing response.

Conversely, I have found that to work in an atmosphere of trust, in groups, and over several days in a residential setting gives people the opportunity to focus entirely on their own healing. In such an environment, clients can let go of everyday stresses and strains, family problems and work worries and, in exploring themselves and their relationship with their illness, gather transformational momentum. Furthermore, over time, groups in a residential setting tend to become greater than the sum of their parts, providing important mutual inspiration, support, focus and a sense of safety.

To further enhance this all-important sense of safety, and therefore increase the depth of exploration possible, my associate and friend, Mary Joan Zakovy and I have developed a kind of "buddy system" for working with patients. By pairing people for integrated bodywork sessions, we have four people in the room at any one time, and have found that the mix of male and female energy and the presence of other people seems to make an environment safe enough for clients to approach what many consider the last taboos — violence and sexuality.

## PHYSICIAN, HEAL THYSELF

It is a truism of psychoanalytic and shamanic practices alike that the healing of the therapeutic relationship is seldom a one-way street: frequently the healer will find herself as challenged, amazed and rewarded as her clients. In my case, the more Mary

Joan and I worked together, the more issues of hidden or re-pressed feelings, and sexuality, came to light for both the clients and ourselves — and I confess with some retrospective wonder-ment that their eruption in treatment came as quite a shock to me. Finally, I was forced to realize that because of the extent of my own sexual wounding I had swept this whole vital area under the rug. It became increasingly evident that the freedom to explore our inner powerlessness and rage, and reclaim sup-pressed sexual energy, was a key to healing — my own as much as my clients'.

Because to allow violence and sexuality in one's patient is to risk allowing or admitting it in oneself, it is perhaps under-standable that finding a "safe" way to explore these most power-ful facets of human experience has eluded almost every healing system to date. But the failure to allow patients to acknowledge them, and the total failure to help patients integrate them, has led many to feel betrayed by our medical profession.

## HONOURING THE MYSTERY

For each of us, the "how" of healing is an unknown. If it were known, of course, we would not be looking for it. Being a totally subjective experience, it defies any objective analysis. Difficult as it may seem, the fact is that each of us must find healing for ourselves, by somehow discovering that innate potential within. Although there are certainly people with experience who can help and guide us on the path, in reality no one can actually perform the deed for someone else. Furthermore, because each person's journey is unique, the specific meaning of someone's symptoms can never be accurately predicted in advance.

Which brings us to the nub of the issue: — *there is a mystery inherent in the healing process which must be accepted and inte-grated as part of the journey.* That mystery reflects the uniqueness of each individual, whose peculiar combination of personality, constitutional strengths or weaknesses, and life situation, can never be fully known. When we try to remove the mystery through rational analysis without reference to the unique individual who is ill — as modern medicine has tried to do — we inadvertently succeed in removing the very thing we are trying to find — healing.

It's quite possible the Zulu woman knew this intuitively but had no way of communicating it to her Western-trained physicians who operated from entirely different assumptions. To them a uterus was a uterus but for her dying was perhaps her only solution. The fact that she was fully willing — even determined — to enter the final void with no chance of return, was something we might do better to honour than dismiss.

And to do that, we might have to question many of our basic assumptions, even enter a kind of void ourselves.

# Chapter 2

# THE VOID:
## threshold to healing

*There is a crack in everything;*
*That's how the light gets in.*

— Leonard Cohen

$O$ ne of the cornerstones of the healing process is the appearance — whether it be sudden or gradual — of a profound attitudinal shift which might best be described as "transformational." However, as we've seen, the shift is much more than a change from one perspective to another. It is rather a shift toward a *positionless position*. As impossible as it may seem, to begin the healing journey we have to discover that non-place within ourselves which I have chosen to refer to in this book as "the void" — a place altogether beyond conflicting perspectives.

As we move across its threshold, our sense of dichotomy (female/male, subject/object, body/mind) and separation which seem so self-evident in our everyday reality recede until finally even the distinction between observer and observed dissolves and uncharted territory seems to explode in all directions.

Here, we enter a whole new world, a world where only being exists, where the underlying energy which is the essence of all things and present in everything around us manifests itself. Here, everything is part of the whole and nothing — including illness — is alien.

## THE WOOD BETWEEN WORLDS

In *The Magician's Nephew*, the first of C.S. Lewis' Narnia chronicles, there was a "wood between the worlds" which led to Narnia. It was a verdant woodland containing numberless small ponds, each of which led to a different world. These ponds acted as doorways, thresholds to somewhere else, rather than as things in themselves.

One of the ponds, for example, led to Earth; another to Narnia; and countless other ponds led to worlds of all kinds. And the ponds were limitless; the choice of worlds limitless. Unknown ponds are described stretching endlessly in all directions, suggesting an infinite variety of possible experiences. But along with the excitement of the unknown lurked its dangers. The wood contained a profound sleepiness which could wipe out memory and prevent a return to Earth; and the worlds accessed through the ponds were uncharted and could be disturbing or even hazardous. Once a visitor entered a pond, there was literally no knowing what would happen!

## THE VOID

Although the Narnia stories were written for children, their suggestive imagery can be just as significant for adults. In the context of the healing journey, we might understand the wood between worlds as a place of possibilities rather than actualities. In many ways it is a state analogous to an infant's consciousness before it acquires the capacity for what we call "pattern recognition." And it is an admirable analogy for the void.

## REALITY AS PATTERN RECOGNITION

"Reality" is whatever it is; but we understand it by recognizing patterns in it according to our cultural training and upbringing. In a sense, then, the void mimics the perception of a newborn, whose eyes register a myriad of visual data but who is not yet capable of making human sense of it. Similarly, the void takes us back to that state prior to "knowledge" and subject-object distinctions which guide us in determining what we are seeing based on what we have seen in the past.

In other words, there is infinite potential and possibility in the void but no *specific* "experience" as we are used to understanding it. That is not to say there is no experience at all, but rather no specific experience. Looked at this way, Lewis' ponds might be thought of as points of entry to, and exit from, the state of infinite and chaotic experiential potential.

The void, then, like those ponds, is both nothing and everything and neither nothing nor everything; both empty and full and yet neither empty nor full, all at the same time. Since it has no particular content, it has the potential for all contents. It is literally brimming with potential, a flexible and malleable "virtual reality" — remarkably like a pond — which can be consciously entered to allow the development of new patterns of understanding and new realities.

When life presents insuperable problems, the void is the place to reassess our situation and discover new ways of being. It is in this place of unlimited possibility that we discover the secrets of healing.

## CONTEXT AND INTENTION

There are two elements which are essential in the use of the void for healing, elements which are perhaps best identified as "context" and "intention." Though these concepts may at first seem unfamiliar, they can be readily understood with reference to the way we use language to communicate. Briefly, "intention" is our desire to express a certain idea while "context" refers to the particular environment in which we express it. Ideally, intention and context, working together symbiotically, sift and structure the infinite variety of words which might emerge from language's potential, or void, at any given point to produce meaning.

Many of the same principles apply to healing, where the void we are seeking is found in the limitless and inchoate gaps in our own consciousness. If our context and intention are congruent with healing at the point of entry to this void, then the subsequent manifestation will reflect our intent and the body's natural healing potential will be activated.

## INTENT AND THE DOCTOR-PATIENT RELATIONSHIP

Because healing is fundamentally a natural bodily process, all things being equal, it should proceed quite smoothly. That health is so elusive even where there is good access to medical care speaks to a distortion of both context and intention in the conventional doctor-patient relationship.

The most common distortion is a *diversion of intent* toward relief of symptoms without consideration of the possibility that these same symptoms, if heeded, might contain a message which would give our symptoms some meaning in the context of our lives. Instead, intention shifts to obliterating these messages from the body-mind while doctor and patient collude in avoiding the deeper issues involved in healing. While such an approach appears compassionate, the effort to relieve symptoms, in fact, generally reflects both parties' need to feel secure and in control.

The second problem is a *shift of context* away from an environment of mutual confidentiality, trust and safety toward mutual mistrust and suspicion, as the physician-patient interaction becomes influenced by the darker side of those same issues of security and control. When such agendas constitute the primary intention of doctor and patient, deep healing is postponed.

## FEAR, TRUST AND RESISTANCE

Creative use of the void for any purpose requires that we trust in the outcome without ever knowing exactly what that outcome will be. Resistance compromises the intent and context of the endeavour which in turn distorts the manifestation from the void and may give the erroneous impression that healing is not possible.

Fear is particularly acute in our first encounters with the void, as the carefully honed control strategies of a lifetime are imperiled by new and sometimes uncomfortable insights and the release of long repressed emotions. For this reason, it is crucial to recognize that resistance is natural and that patiently working through it can take some time. For if we absolutely refuse to put our defences aside, deep healing will be blocked.

## ENTERING THE VOID

As readers may have witnessed in reading first pages of this book, descriptions of the void can make it sound formidably complex and full of impenetrable paradoxes. Fortunately, it is a state much simpler to experience than to describe. In fact, nodes of access to the void are everywhere in our daily life if we know where to look for them.

How can we recognize these "ponds," or points of access? They exist in the gaps between things, in the space between activities. Just as a vibrating string contains points of rest which form an essential part of its dynamic system, these nodes are "zero" points, or places of rest in our perception of our constantly active and manifesting reality. Such "gaps" in a dynamic sequence are moments when manifestation falls back into potential, as though into its resting state.

Like any other skill, accessing the void requires practice, but can be learned by anyone who is interested and can be applied to almost any endeavour — whether it be public speaking, cooking breakfast, or healing the body. In fact, most of us are already acquainted with experiences of it in our everyday lives. A brief description of some of these situations follows.

## HYPNOGOGIA AND HYPNOPOMPIA

Every night when we go to sleep, and every morning when we wake up, we pass from the rational world into the subjective, or dream world, and back again. The void can be accessed between these two states. As we pass from one state of consciousness to another, we pass through a narrow gap which constitutes the transition between waking and sleeping. Those spaces are nodal points — doorways to the void — which have been variously termed "hypnogogia" (falling asleep) and "hypnopompia" (waking up).

In these somnolent spaces, inner and outer begin to merge with each other, resulting in an experience of identity without a fixed observable reality. From the point of view of the objective rational world, the dream world is unreal, unfocused, non-linear and unimportant. When we wake up, it recedes and virtually disappears. But the reverse is also true. From the point of view of the dream world, the world of everyday reality appears unreal and unimportant while the dream world holds sway. In the void, we are not fully in a dream nor are we fully awake but somewhere between the two, with conscious access to both states though not fully present in either.

It's possible, with relatively little practice, to stay somnolent for quite a while before completely waking up. Indeed, the hypnopompic state is so easy to achieve that virtually everyone is familiar with it. Few people however, are aware of hypnopompia's immense significance in healing. It is here, in this half-awake state that we can bring dreams to consciousness and begin to explore the no-man's-land that lies between our rational and irrational minds.

## MEDITATION

Those people who meditate will be even more familiar with the void. Because meditation is an effective way to bring the mind to a resting state, it can be a conscious and formal way of entering the void on a regular basis. During meditation, the external sensual world recedes and attention shifts to the inner world. Sometimes even the inner world recedes and only the sense of being remains. In that state of mindfulness, the inner and outer are experienced simultaneously in such a way that they can be integrated.

Interestingly, some meditation techniques encourage meditating at dawn and dusk, precisely because those times represent nodal points between day and night, points which mark a transition in our experience of our world.

## GUIDED HYPERVENTILATION

Increased breathing shifts attention from the outer to the inner world, from the rational to the irrational, from the mind to the body and beyond. Hyperventilation can be a powerful way of entering the void but is best done under supervision. Occasionally, disorientation can persist for some time afterward and interfere with the intellect's usual mode of functioning in the world. Practised in a retreat setting, with people familiar with the technique, it can be a quick and effective way to permit deep encounters with the void.

While hyperventilation can be effortful initially, the need for effort recedes as the void is accessed and awareness of the breath becomes an anchor of safety in a sea of chaos and fear. Both under- and over-breathing can prevent access to the void and may reflect the natural resistance the ego has to letting go of control. Discovery of the void is very much like finding one's balance point on a gymnastics beam. It may seem difficult initially but, once there, breathing can be used as a kind of internal balancing pole, permitting maintenance of the altered state. As with any skill, practice and persistence generally get results.

## ACUPUNCTURE

Acupuncture is another potent way to explore the void and is well suited to assisting many aspects of an exploration of mind/body/spirit. It seems to work very well in tandem with guided hyperventilation to catapult eager travellers into the deeper reaches of the void. Indeed, it can facilitate appropriate breathing in such a way that almost no effort is required to engage the process. I have seen acupuncture so effective on occasion that the insertion of a single needle is sometimes all that is necessary to open the doorway to the void.

One branch of acupuncture, the so-called "5-element" acupuncture, is particularly effective because it targets the personality rather than symptomatology. According to the 5-element model, we are all born with individual natures which primarily emulate the quality of energy present in a particular season. Over time, this energy becomes compromised as we conform our behaviour to "fit in" with familial or societal expectations and pain or illness may result.

The choice of acupuncture points according to constitutional type, then, can help people rediscover their natural way of being. By focusing on the person rather than the symptom, it effectively shifts intention away from symptom control toward integrating the total body/mind/spirit. In doing so, it provides a context for the patient's entry into the void which is congruent with healing.

## RETREATS

Ultimately, everybody wants to be loved and accepted for who they really are. Of course, only when we can do it for ourselves can we say that our healing has been truly internalized. The unconditional love which the therapeutic situation strives for is modelled on the ideal parental relationship. Unfortunately for many, such love is viewed with intense suspicion as their personal experience may have been of love given or withheld manipulatively, as an instrument of power and control.

In practice, the development of the trust which is so crucial to the healing relationship requires a sustained atmosphere of acceptance for every person's uniqueness. That generally takes time, patience and non-judgemental attention to the particular character, fears and perspectives of each individual. Therefore, as mentioned in the last chapter, a residential setting can, by providing these essentials to trust, facilitate a deep and extremely powerful experience of the void and strongly promote the healing response.

## GROUPS

Working in a group situation can greatly facilitate a deep inner exploration. When a number of people are gathered together for the purposes of healing, a fruitful rapport is usually achieved much more quickly than in the conventional doctor-patient relationship, which is often fraught with unacknowledged power struggles. Furthermore, the experience of working in a group can be such a different experience for many people that it constitutes a "gap" in their lives, a gap which — almost by definition — can be a void experience.

## THE HEALER PHENOMENON

The healer phenomenon has always excited much interest. It seems that certain people have the gift of healing in their hands — sometimes in their very presence. What are they doing, if anything?

In my view, successful healers, whether they are conscious of it or not, locate their awareness in the void when they work.

Their intention is to heal rather than to relieve symptoms and they appreciate each individual's uniqueness. In addition, they trust that the outcome of any particular interaction will be appropriate, and are therefore detached as to its particular form. That is why many healers will say they are "not doing anything," or claim that they are merely acting as a "channel," that a greater power is working through them.

By placing their consciousness in the void, healers encourage us to enter a similar space. In that way, we discover our own inner healer quite spontaneously and take charge of our own healing process.

When we consciously enter the void for the purposes of healing, the body-mind and spirit can speak to us in new — and ultimately wonderful — ways. In many cases, the result can be a total and profound transformation of our relationship to ourselves, our illness and the world.

Chapter 3

# POWER AND THE GUARDIAN

*Where love rules, there is no will to power, and where power predominates, there love is lacking. The one is the shadow of the other.*

— Carl Jung

*I*t is my view that when we are ill we are not helpless at all but rather deny our own power, willfully blinding ourselves to our own strength; and, further, that it is this blindness to our true nature that is ultimately what illness is. What our society as a whole cannot face — personal integrity and responsibility — individuals are compelled to grapple with when ill.

The power of the medical establishment is based on our collective insistence that the physician control our sickness, as though it were a distinct and external phenomenon. Our fear of illness — our fear of loss of control — seems, paradoxically, to leave us craving a system that will corroborate our own denial of our power.

But when we talk about our "power," we must be sure we know what we are talking about, for there is a very great difference between the *ability to control* and deep resources of *inner strength* — either of which can be termed "power." The abrogation of the ill individual's inner strength in the Western medical model of doctor-patient relationships seems clearly intended but is perhaps not fully understood or acknowledged.

Where has the power gone, if we don't feel we have it?

## THE GATES OF HADES

In Greek mythology, the gates to the realm of Hades, Lord of the Underworld, were guarded by a frightening three-headed dog called Cerberus. He would let the dead enter but once past his gnashing teeth and spiked tail, they could never get out again. The seeming power of that threatening beast repelled all but the bravest of living souls. Few ventured voluntarily into Hades' kingdom; and those who did were forever changed by their experience. Most were too frightened even to wander near the gates.

Tackling such an apparently awesome power is central to healing. If the experience of illness makes us feel vulnerable and helpless — at the mercy of both the illness and the medical establishment — the healing process must include a retrieval of power and a sense of being in control of our experience.

While this idea may be attractive in theory, however, fear of *dis*ease (pain or illness) is written into the very fabric of our psyches and of modern medicine. Our health care system seems to function on the implicit assumption that patients are helpless "victims" dependent on the all-knowing and all-powerful doctor.

Taking personal control in such a situation can be terrifying. And the resistance to conscious confrontation of one's disease is exactly comparable to the ancients' fear of Cerberus and the descent into Hades, from which they had been led to believe no one returned. Like it or not, however, we must venture deeply into illness to find health and wholeness. And when eventually we cross the threshold and confront our worst fears, we will be forever changed by the experience.

## MARIE: CHRONIC LYMPHATIC LEUKAEMIA

Some time ago, I saw a woman with chronic lymphatic leukaemia which had been diagnosed two years previously. Because the condition was only slowly progressive, her physicians decided there was no need for treatment until symptoms — easy bruising, fatigue from anaemia, or susceptibility to infections from deterioration in immune function — developed. Marie had been advised to go home and get on with her life. Her illness would be monitored with regular white blood cell counts.

Although such an approach seemed entirely reasonable to her physicians, Marie was devastated. She felt she had a death sentence hanging over her head, and no one was willing to do anything about it. She was angry and hostile, and blamed the physicians who had informed her she had the disease.

"I'd rather they hadn't told me anything," she raged during our first meeting, "...though of course I firmly believe in my right to be fully informed."

I could sympathize with the double bind she was in but didn't want to be the next target of her helpless outrage. Her understandable anger was being unleashed onto anyone and everyone, in a determined attempt to deny her personal power. "Inform everyone but me," she seemed to be saying, "because I just don't want to know."

It seems we deny our power and project it onto others out of fear. Though this is partly a result of learned helplessness from childhood, the tragedy is that as adults we waste energy fighting to regain — or even to have acknowledged — *the very power we ourselves have given away.*

This is precisely where Marie found herself. After her diagnosis of leukaemia she felt powerless and controlled. All her available energy was sucked into an impotent rage. And the angrier she became at her helplessness, the higher went her white cell count.

WHO — OR WHAT — IS ILL?

The idea that personal power might be wilfully shunned — as an integral aspect of being ill — is not a conclusion I have come to lightly. Rather, the practice of medicine has led me to the uncomfortable insight that illness is often unconsciously used to bolster a denial of personal responsibility. And when society as a whole supports this denial, it reflects a colossal collective denial.

To point this out and, worse, to appear to blame the ill for their illnesses, is not really socially acceptable. Society, in much the same way as Marie, just "doesn't want to know." Unfortunately, such insistence on their victimization is usually the single most important barrier to patients' finding their way back to health. That our health care systems actively support this situation is a cruel irony, because it perpetuates pain and illness in many people who could otherwise get on with their lives.

## RECONNECTING WITH OUR INNER STRENGTH

Just as many traditional societies challenged and honoured their maturing youths with frightening and demanding rituals focused on confirming their inner strengths, modern societies might choose to challenge their collective immaturity — typified by our refusal of personal power — by turning to face the fearsome monster we have made of bodily pain and illness. If we cannot do this, I believe we will continue to live in a Peter Pan society. Sooner or later, our collective resources will evaporate, and we will face the dilemma of who will rescue whom.

Retrieving personal power involves disillusionment, a deliberate disenchantment with the external forces we've come to depend on. In one sense, the decision to look in a different direction is the first step away from the safety of the known, the comfort of the parental figure of medicine. We enter a world which is both terrifying and creative.

For those who are healthy, this turning away can be intuitive, or perhaps a matter of simple curiosity. For those with chronic illness the choice may be more urgent. Since by definition medicine has failed in chronic illness, our belief in a physician's healing power is a woeful reflection of our sense of our own utter helplessness. So why not follow our own path? Who says we have to do what a doctor tells us when illness presents us with a unique opportunity to engage in the transformational journey of individuation.

So let's explore. Understanding how power operates, we can dismantle it, and perhaps move on to a new and enabled, authentic way of being.

## POWER AS CONTROL

Power can be defined as the capacity to control events in the external world. We generally like to be in control, and dislike feeling helpless. Most of us learned coping strategies of one kind or another to control everything we could very early on in life — with the result that we live driven by a nagging insecurity we have never stopped to decipher.

Coping strategies are an example of the kind of power which is directed away from the self. Its purpose seems to be to expose us to minimal perceptible risk from the outside world. Through such strategies of control we try to force the universe to conform to our needs without demanding anything from us in return. And we expect to feel secure to the degree to which we have succeeded in this — without recognizing that if our motive is an avoidance of helplessness and we are acting out of fear of that helplessness, we are in fact totally controlled by that fear. *When we need to control, we are in turn controlled by that need.* And to be controlled puts us right back in the position of helplessness which we sought to avoid by seeking control.

But when science turns human beings into ciphers, self-knowledge is replaced by statistical analyses. Briefly, the fundamental Cartesian bias our society embraced some two or three hundred years ago is this: our perception of "our" world delivers facts. Put another way, the observer is utterly distinct from what she/he observes.

This bias has produced such jewels of disempowerment as the "randomized double-blind research trial," which purports to test the efficacy of treatment regimens delivered to a radically generalized or generic — human being. Such mass trials — requiring expert interpretation of their data, and carefully preserving their authority by writing off unusual results as "anomalies" — have ingrained deferral of authority to an outside agency in our medical system to the point that individual therapeutic relationships are utterly dehumanized.

When a mass trial purports to show the value of one form of treatment over another, then one treatment of a particular disease becomes right, and any other wrong or inferior, in whatever situation. Power which has already been transferred from patient to physician, now resides with the scientist, leaving the physician as a mere interpreter of distant expertise and diligent student of trial results and "correct" treatment regimens.

This sort of right/wrong thinking can only leave everyone, doctor and patient alike, feeling victimized. Obliged to practise according to certain protocols, physicians feel they must recommend "evidence-based" treatments, and avoid unconventional or "unproven" (albeit perhaps millennia-old) techniques, even though the accepted treatment regimens may have undesirable side-effects. And if power is external, then someone else must be at fault when something goes wrong. When those side-effects arise, as they inevitably must, someone other than the patient has to be held responsible, even though it was the patient who decided to take the treatment. The plethora of medical malpractice suits attests to the devastation this approach can bring.

To suggest one form of treatment is good for all people in all situations seems patently absurd. Yet physicians have allowed fear to provoke them to abandon their inner strength and intuition and relinquish their authority when dealing with patients.

## POWER AS STRENGTH

Power exercised over others as control, or projected onto authority figures and then vehemently contested is quite different from power accepted as one's own. Whereas control is reactive and manipulative, strength can be defined as the potential to act effectively.

Individuals who trust themselves to deal with any situation which arises can be said to have inner strength. They understand that real power may manifest as an ability to surrender to the moment. They see no need to control events but accept and learn from what comes their way.

## POWER AND THE DOCTOR/PATIENT RELATIONSHIP

The traditional therapeutic relationship is deliberately one of mutual dependence. People acquire a doctor on whom they feel they can rely, and family physicians acquire a list of patients who they "look after"; and each believes they need the other.

Such an arrangement seems only sensible. Illness is so unpredictable, we argue, it's reasonable to have a family doctor who will help out in bad times. And that is certainly true for those rare occasions when catastrophe strikes. The difficulty is that most illnesses do not strike us out of the blue as we would like to believe, but are the predictable result of years of imbalanced living and a vigorous suppression of warning signals.

Unfortunately, modern medicine is ill-equipped to address the epidemic of psychosomatic anxiety in our society which is proving so devastating to our health. As the term "psychosomatic" ("psyche" being mind; "soma," body) indicates, such illness is a condition of the mind and spirit as well as the body — a spiritual malaise — and the bandaid medicine it attracts is a denial of the real meaning of health.

At the same time, the balance of power in the relationship between physicians and patients is shifting. We have made health a product to be bought and sold. And consumer power and advocacy is at an all-time high. Many Western countries enjoy unlimited free medical care, and the right to sue physicians. So, while doctors may be seen as having enormous, life-giving power, those same physicians fear their patients' *life-denying* power — the power, in other words, to deprive them of their livelihood.

Mighty powers indeed. Who then is really in control? Both, and neither. Because each thinks the other has such great power, each lives in fear of the other, denying their own innate inner strength. Such relationships rarely lead to healing.

## STRENGTH IN THE THERAPEUTIC RELATIONSHIP

Nothing much of any import occurs when both parties are operating from control, because their fear straightjackets any desire for radical change. When we retrieve our own power, however, the nature of all our relationships changes dramatically and a true "healing journey" may be undertaken.

The first step is perhaps the most difficult of the whole healing journey. We all must face Cerberus alone: crossing Hades' threshold is mandatory for any deeper work to begin. Obviously, the physician has the primary responsibility to take that first step as an example, but it is incumbent on the client to take a similar step early in the relationship, or no further movement will take place. The crucial thing is that we must all take the first step on our own, without knowing if it is safe to do so.

I remember one man with chronic headaches who spent ten days with us in a residential program and who adamantly refused to let anyone touch him the whole time he was there. While we respected his wishes and left him alone, stopping only to talk to him and interact as much as he would permit, when he left us he complained our therapy had made him worse! Such is the power of projection.

Once bitten twice shy, it would seem, and many chronic sufferers have felt so betrayed by the medical establishment that they are loathe to trust again. But shy or not we must risk reaching out if we are ever to heal. Waiting to feel safe because all we have ever experienced is betrayal of trust can leave us waiting for ever. Healing involves a change, and change requires change.

The fearsome animal guarding the gates to the realm of the soul exactly mirrors the defences and the fear surrounding this first step into the void. Before entering the void, we must pass that fiercely defended threshold, and befriend the creature which guards it. When we do, the first glimmer of our inner strength returns. The power of the guardian is the fear of ourselves. By facing the guardian, not only do we acquire its power but it becomes our ally and our strength.

## MARIE'S JOURNEY: SYMPTOMS AND SOUL LOSS

Fortunately, Marie's journey had a brave and hopeful beginning. Two years of feeling powerless had left her ready to explore her rage and acknowledge her strength. Her anger bubbled to the surface like lava and it was only a matter of giving her permission for her to make a connection between her feelings and her leukaemia. At that point, she boldly stepped over the threshold and was on her way.

The symptom, seen as a marker of denial or grief, can be used as a pointer to the lost or denied aspect of an individual's soul. And if this is so, then the business of healing is a business of the soul, and the ultimate goal of healing is not simply the relief of symptoms but the recovery — or recognition — of our inner strength and support for our transformational journeys.

# Chapter 4

# NAMING :
## dismantling the illusion of power

*Remember the false self is false; it is non-existent, but by believing in it, we act as if it were real.*

— Vernon Howard

*H*ow can we free ourselves from the disempowering spell of the conventional medical establishment's "Aesculapian authority" — a disempowerment radically incompatible with real healing? And how can we move toward a therapeutic relationship based instead on mutual respect, trust and courage?

There is no simple answer to such questions because illness nearly always indicates that we have lost some measure of our inner strength, and that loss is a significant part of the illness. In fact, illness and loss of inner strength appear together so frequently one could say that they are really different aspects of the same thing.

Consequently, then, any medicine which does not assist us to recover our inner strength and fails to teach us how to look after ourselves in the end only creates a self-serving dependency — or to be frank, a co-dependency. Though we may seem to get well from such treatment, in fact the root imbalance will remain and we will configure new illnesses, one after another, until either death or true healing occurs. In this way, our present system of medicine actually betrays us while appearing to help.

However, Aesculapian authority — like many other kinds of authority — is based on the fact that its workings are unexamined. It caves in once exposed to the light of full consciousness. Still, changing the system will do little because, as we have seen in the previous chapter, as long as individual doctors and patients remain powerless, the therapeutic relationship will be the way it is. Real change, then, can only happen from within ourselves.

One familiar story which speaks to this issue is the tale of Rumpelstiltskin.

## RUMPELSTILTSKIN

There once was a poor miller who lived alone with his only child, a daughter. One day, when the daughter was nearly grown, the miller took her to see the King; and to impress him, told the King that the young woman could weave straw into gold. Now, the King was very fond of gold and he said to the miller, "That is a talent which would please me well. If your daughter is so very clever, bring her again to the castle tomorrow and we will see what she can do."

As soon as she arrived, the King led the miller's daughter into a chamber full of straw; and he gave her a wheel and a reel saying, "Now set to work, for if you have not spun this straw into gold by dawn tomorrow, you must die." With these words he locked her in the room and left her alone.

And there the miller's poor daughter sat; and she sat for a long, long time for of course she had no idea how to spin straw into gold. And as she sat, wondering how to save her life, her grief and terror grew. Eventually, she began to weep.

Then all at once, the door the King had locked behind him sprang open and into the room stepped a little man who said, "Good evening, fair maiden, why do you weep?"

"Ah," she replied, "there is no help for me, for I must spin this straw into gold, or die."

"What will you give me if I spin it for you?" asked the little man.

"The necklace from my neck," said the miller's daughter.

And so the Dwarf set to work. He placed himself in front of the wheel and filled first one bobbin, then two, then three; all night long he worked, until every bobbin was full of gold. Then, without a word, he took the necklace and left.

Not long after, the King came in and was very much astonished to see the glistening bobbins. But though the sight gladdened him it made his heart more greedy yet; and he led the miller's daughter into another larger room, also full of straw, and bade her spin it into gold during the night if she valued her life. The young woman was again quite at a loss as to what to do. But while she cried — perhaps a little expectantly this time — the locked door was flung open as before and the Dwarf appeared and again asked her what she would give him in return for his help.

"The ring off my finger," she replied.

So the little man took the ring and began to spin and by morning all the straw was gold. The King again rejoiced at the sight but still he was not sated. Showing the girl a still larger room full of straw, he said, "All this you must spin this night; and if you succeed you shall be my bride," and left thinking what a wealthy monarch he was going to be.

Again the Dwarf appeared, asking, "What will you give me?"

"I have nothing left," confessed the miller's daughter.

"Then promise me your first-born child when you become queen," he said.

"Who can tell if that will ever happen?" the miller's daughter thought; and, not knowing how else to help herself, she promised the Dwarf what he asked. The little man set to as before and at length finished the spinning. When morning came and the King found all he desired, he celebrated his wedding; and so the miller's daughter became queen.

About a year after her marriage, when she had forgotten all about the Dwarf, the Queen brought a fine child into the world.

Sure enough, soon after its birth, the little man appeared and demanded his wages. Aghast, the young Queen offered him all the riches of her kingdom. But the Dwarf answered: "No, wealth I do not need; it's the child I want."

Then the Queen began to weep and groan so much that the Dwarf pitied her and said, "I will give you three days. If in that time you discover what my name is, you shall keep your son."

So, all night the Queen racked her brains; and before dawn she sent messengers far and wide collecting every name in the kingdom. The following morning, the Dwarf came and she began guessing with "Peter," "John," "Bartholomew," trying all the names she knew. But each time the little man replied, "That is not my name." The second day, the Queen's criers in all of her villages sang out to her people for curious names; and she called the Dwarf to her and told him every one, but still he replied, "That is not my name."

The third day a messenger she had sent abroad came back and said: "I have not found a single new name; but I came to a high mountain near the edge of the forest where I saw a little house; and before the door a fire was burning, and 'round the fire a very curious little man was dancing on one leg and shouting:

> *Today I stew, and then I'll bake,*
> *Tomorrow I shall the Queen's child take;*
> *There's no doubt the wager I'll win*
> *'Cause my name is Rumpelstiltskin.*

When the Queen heard this story she was very glad, for now she knew the name. Soon after, the Dwarf came to her and asked, "Now, my lady Queen, it is your last day, what is my name?"

She mentioned a couple of ordinary names to make him feel at ease, and then said, "Are you called Rumpelstiltskin?"

"A witch has told you!" the little man shrieked, stamping his right foot on the ground so hard it stuck fast, whereupon he pulled it so hard that his right hand came off, and he hopped away, howling terribly. And from that day to this the Queen has heard no more from her troublesome visitor.

## HER STORY, OUR STORY

One of many ways of interpreting the vast richness of traditional stories is to understand each character as a representation of a part of our psyche. In the tale of Rumpelstiltskin, then, we might understand the King to represent our ego, or rational consciousness, while the miller's daughter could be said to represent our emotional body or feeling. The miller himself might be our superego, or "inner parent," and the Dwarf might represent a challenge or threat to which we must respond. Finally, the royal couple's infant signifies our potential to create new life through the integration of fragmented wholes: in other words, to create a new wholeness, or to find healing.

This reading of the story shows us a circumstance in which the superego (the miller) is willing to put the life of the emotional body — represented by his only child — at risk to satisfy its own ambitions. The story further suggests that the miller understands that in order to sell the King on his daughter's worth, he must pitch her value in terms the King will understand. He seems to know that the ego (the King) is insatiably greedy and misunderstands the true worth of the psyche's emotional nature. The King views the young woman only as a means to his ends — in this case, greater and greater worldly power — and allows her into his castle only to exploit her.

It is striking how little concern the King appears to have for the girl, valuing only the gold he imagines she produces. It is also striking how very uneasy she seems to make him. It is as though the ego lets feeling into its fortress only to immediately lock her in a remote room, threatening to kill her if she does not do exactly as he expects.

Further, it's clear the King doesn't understand how straw is turned to gold, nor does he care; but he does understand gold. No sooner has one batch been spun than he wants more and, night after night, the miller's daughter has to spin ever larger amounts for her greedy suitor. But of course, the task is not humanly possible — no matter how large or small the amount — and so the girl to save her life must barter first her own meager possessions and finally her future.

And so it goes. The miller tempts the King, and the King demands of his daughter, and she in turn must bargain with the Dwarf, who offers his services — for a price. In much the same way, it seems, we are inclined to sacrifice our life-force for our material wellbeing, if not outright greed, and value our feeling nature for what it can give us.

## DEFICIENT QI: THE PRINCE'S RANSOM

As financial security becomes more elusive in our society, many people must sacrifice more and more to get it, ending up on a treadmill which drains their energy and morbidly dampens their spirits. It is no wonder that practitioners of Chinese Traditional Medicine note that the predominant energetic configuration in the West is a low energy condition known as "Deficient Qi."

The Dwarf represents the kind of threat many of us feel and the kind of bargain many of us make, offering all that we have — and more — to meet our ego's (and our superego's) demands and ambitions. Most commonly, we take wages in return for soul-destroying work. And find, as does the miller's daughter, that as the demands from the ego grow more and more exorbitant, so too do the demands of the Dwarf until we are paying not only with our present resources but with our futures: in fact, with our very lives.

The Dwarf exacts a bigger price each time he shows up to help out, until eventually the miller's daughter is forced to sell her unborn child to meet the King's demands. The sacrifice of our potential for the sake of the ego's security, the story seems to tell us, is a Faustian bargain which damages the heart.

## SELLING OUT THE SOUL

Consider what we have learned. A young woman is shut up in a room and commanded to fulfil increasingly exorbitant and inhuman tasks on pain of death in what turns out to be a weird kind of courtship ritual. And her talent — the talent the King wants to own — is an imaginary one. In fact, it belongs to the Dwarf to whom she has quite literally sold herself in order to survive.

It is an ugly scene: the King who was already rich enough becomes richer at the expense of the peasant girl; and she, who was already his subject, becomes his slave; and is eventually forced to sell her unborn child — or, we might say, her inner strength. As far as the intellect is concerned, it seems, life energy and feeling are only valuable for the material wellbeing or status they can produce. They have no value in and of themselves.

Ugly — but perhaps all too familiar?

## CHANCE DISCOVERY OF THE NAME

Normally, this misuse or suppression of the feminine principle becomes increasingly costly to body and soul until illness interrupts. But this is not how our present story ends. If we continue our analogy, we see that the miller's daughter's future is jeopardized only until she discovers the real identity of the "little man" to whom she has indebted herself. We should also note that she discovers this name only after a desperate — and ultimately fruitless — three-day search "all over her kingdom." At the last moment, in a seemingly chance encounter, the power which has almost stolen her future life *gives its own identity away.*

Now what could the act of naming have to do with a retrieval of inner strength? How can knowing and speaking a name give the soul its freedom? And what has it got to do with health?

Physicians are often admonished to be very careful what they say to patients because their words carry enormous weight. Few patients ever question their authority or that of the medical system. And because power can also gull itself, doctors themselves too often fall for the myth of Aesculapian authority and are trapped as surely as any of their patients in a belief in their own godlike powers. But when things go wrong, those same patients feel betrayed, and may hold their physicians or the medical system responsible.

The Dwarf in the story of Rumpelstiltskin might be said to represent the kind of power we give our physicians. "Only give your all to me," the Dwarf invites us, "and all will be well." Little do we understand what we are giving away. As long as we displace responsibility for health onto our physicians, we remain distanced from our own inner resources, the potential we all have to heal from within.

As a society, we've no idea how damaging this is. Patients come to a physician to find healing but in misunderstanding the identity of the physician and his or her powers, we sacrifice a crucial relationship to our own inner strength. The one really important aspect of healing — the recovery of the soul — is denied us.

## CALLING OUT THE NAME

Rumpelstiltskin sounds like a nonsense name. An English-speaker listening to the tale may understand that calling it notifies the Dwarf that the game is up; that his game is "nonsense." But a German-speaking listener — for whom the tale was originally intended — might hear something else. In Rumpelstiltskin are suggestions of "rumble" and "topsy-turvy" but also of "still" or "quiet" and "child" or "baby." So it may be that what the Queen says, at the last minute, and just in time, when confronted by her tormentor is, "I am silencing the rumblings of my child" or, in plain English, "I am not listening to myself." In other words, as we hinted at the beginning of the chapter, it is the awareness of the illusion of power which neutralizes that power. When we realize that it is we ourselves who have sold ourselves into another's power, we begin to regain our inner strength.

With the destruction of illusions comes the potential for new understanding and insight. Physician and patient may both need to be released from the bargains they've made with their "dwarfs" and call their powers by their correct names. So long as either hangs onto a belief in inhuman powers or false authority, they will remain in the grip of their illusions and pay for it with their health and strength.

But release may not come without a fight. At the time of naming, disillusionment may produce anger. At hearing himself named, the Dwarf — who after all represents part of our own psyche — literally tears himself limb from limb and stomps away in rage. We may feel very angry at being duped for so long and we may want to strike out at anyone who happens to be around rather than realize we are angry at our own naïveté. It is a dangerous phase: the released energy can be destructive. But if we can negotiate the minefield, we are free to move on.

When both patient and physician can admit their real natures and name their illusions and human limitations, they are released from the Dwarf's power. Physicians are released from the need to pretend they know what to do, or to diagnose and treat what they cannot entirely understand — and patients can reclaim their own authority and learn to honour their own intuitions and hunches. Both are freed to follow whatever direction seems appropriate to the needs of the moment; and at that point, true healing can begin.

Part II

SPIRIT

*and*

THE ROOT OF ILLNESS

## Chapter 5

# THE DESCENT OF SPIRIT

*If you bring forth that which is within you,*
*That which is within you will save you.*
*If you do not bring forth that which is within you,*
*That which is within you will destroy you.*

— The Gospel of St. Thomas

*J*oe was a twenty-five-year-old artist who was frequently ill with chest infections. He smoked twenty cigarettes a
day even though he knew he shouldn't and was never able to
stop for more than a day or two before his anxiety would force
him to light up again. He had never been in the best of health —
even as a child he had been listless and susceptible to coughs,
colds and ear infections.

"Why do you keep smoking?" I asked him when he was ill
with pneumonia for the umpteenth time.

"I don't know, Doc," he told me. "I've tried to quit but I can't.
Sometimes I think my smokes are the only friends I've got."

Some friends, I thought. Here was a young man with a
weak constitution who was suffering from repeated lung infections. His smoking was clearly jeopardizing his health and he
knew it but felt he couldn't stop because of his nervous loneliness. Yet the "cause" of his illness according to my training was
streptococcus and the "cure" was penicillin.

"What utter nonsense," I used to think without having a
clue what to do about it. Such an obvious example of the limitations of the cause and effect model used to rile me in my early
practice yet it was many years before I could begin to see what
was really going on.

Streptococcus was less the real cause of Joe's pneumonia than it was a convenient scapegoat which enabled him to carry on his denial of his real dis-ease. And by treating him with penicillin, I was colluding in that denial by addressing only the bacteria. The fact was that Joe's constitutional weakness was inseparable from his low spirits which in turn promoted his self-destructive habit and predisposed him to lung disease. He was bound to get pneumonia sooner or later, and get it again and again.

My experience with Joe and many others like him when I was in general practice gradually deepened my intuitive understanding of the body-mind-spirit continuum and its implications for healing. Today, I wonder how modern medicine can possibly maintain such a drastically limited view of the causes of illness.

## HEALING THE BODY-MIND-SPIRIT

Conventional medicine tends to separate the mind from the body and refuses to consider the spirit at all. However, if illness first manifests at the level of the spirit, this reductive view of human life is part of the problem of illness.

What does it mean to take a "body-mind-spirit" approach to healing? Though I have misgivings about the phrase body-mind-spirit — which might be seen to perpetuate our perception of our beingness as threefold rather than as a unity — it is intended to denote the undifferentiated totality of our being and to imply a holistic understanding of several integrated levels of wellness and illness in which neither mind (the beliefs of the Zulu woman, for example) nor spirit (Joe's loneliness) can be ignored.

Let's look at these interrelated areas for a moment.

## SPIRIT

It can seem nearly impossible to talk about "spirit" in the singular without conjuring up religious traditions of one kind or another. But if we can fuse this larger understanding of spirit with our more everyday sense of having high or low *spirits* — being exuberant, happy and energetic, or negative, lethargic and depressed — we can perhaps grasp one important aspect of the meaning of spirit inherent in the phrase body-mind-spirit.

Our spirits rise naturally when the soul is fully expressed and the life current is flowing without hindrance. We can only know the soul by expressing it, and when we do that, our spirits rise spontaneously. Much like the carpenter's tool of the same name, our "spirit level" — the measure of our spirit — can be a measure of our overall balance. When we are expressing our full potential, we feel good about living. It's that simple.

It is also our spirit which links us to the life force in everything around us, the vital energies which know no physical boundaries. Our spirit has an inborn understanding of a fundamental unity in phenomena which some have termed the "big-S" Self, or "world soul," as opposed to the "small-s" self or ego. If we think and act in ways that disallow that understanding we betray a very real part of our own selves and our being in the world.

MIND

The intellect, as Claude Lévi-Strauss long ago pointed out, works by opposition and tends to see in terms of dualities, of choices, and of opposing and often contradictory possibilities. The intellect chooses between this or that, right or wrong, black or white, good or bad.

There is nothing inherently wrong with choosing and distinguishing. Indeed since no choice is still a choice, we have little option but to choose from moment to moment. The mind carries on distinguishing and choosing regardless — just because it is a mind. To maintain optimum health, however, it must acknowledge and allow for the spirit's more holistic understanding — for when the mind imagines that its distinctions have some absolute value, the spirit suffers. Without an awareness of the spirit, the intellect is rootless and swells with self-importance. Mind comes to consider itself the centre of its universe, the individual being. From this vantage point, what cannot be spoken or seen — the spirit — appears as a direct threat. And so the rational mind participates in life by criticizing and moralizing, suppressing aspects of the self — and the "big-S" Self — it deems unacceptable.

This "mistake of the intellect," which is Faust's mistake, and which the early Greeks called *hubris*, reflects an imbalance between mind and spirit. It is the manifestation of an alienation from the larger Self, or universal spirit. Indeed, such a mistake is described in many religious traditions as the root of ignorance and evil and is considered the prelude to disaster — whether societal or individual.

And there are consequences at the physical level, too. The ego-driven efforts of the intellect to maintain itself as king of its castle require that it maintain a constant "armour" against contradictory feeling or experience. This physical and psychological armouring demands a huge expenditure of energy and results in chronic mental and emotional stress and muscular tension which over time produces physical deterioration and degenerative or stress-related diseases.

## THE MOCK BATTLE

The tragedy is that all this struggle is unnecessary. The world is full of contradictions and paradoxes and we need not waste our energy trying to establish the rightness of any one particular point of view. Even science has had to acknowledge — through struggling with the problem of the wave-particle duality inherent in our perception of light — that the more we fix on one aspect of a phenomena, the more we will lose sight of others. We literally see what we want to see, or what we expect to see.

If we remember that the intellect acts as a fairly drastic filter of the complex data our senses deliver to it, then, we will understand that perceived "contradictions" are merely a reminder of its inability to appreciate phenomena in their entirety and thus reflect nothing more or less than our own limitations. Unfortunately, throughout the modern era we have had the arrogance to assume that what we perceived was "what is."

And not only do our minds sift incoming physical data, they also screen our spirits' expressions. By allowing or disallowing their various manifestations, mind acts as a kind of filter for our souls' limitless possibilities, thus producing the coherent and reasonably constant personas we use to function in the world. Unfortunately, this seemingly benign "filter" can as easily distort the soul material being expressed as it can the incoming sensory information — with the inevitable consequences to our health.

BODY

Modern medicine describes illness at the physical level only. Patients like Joe, who for their own reasons also wish to understand illness as a physical phenomenon, generally present physical symptoms — fatigue, pain, infection and so on — around which they can be sure their physician will make a diagnosis which maintains the illusion of physical cause. (Even psychiatry, the branch of medicine which ostensibly concerns itself with the mind, rarely goes beyond the physical model, blaming mental illness on altered brain chemistry and addressing symptoms with drugs.)

Treatment of illness at the level of the body may change the kind of illnesses we get but it does not alter the fact that we will get ill; and it does not encourage wellness. Treating Joe's pneumonia with antibiotics did not make Joe well. In fact, because it allowed him to put off facing the consequences of his behaviour, it in fact maintained him in an unhealthy state.

## ILLNESS AS "DESCENT OF SPIRIT"

A profound way of understanding illness is to see it as a "precipitate" of denied spiritual material, or, to use Alfred Ziegler's phrase, a "spiritual descent." When soul material is habitually held back, the inner tension which builds in the body eventually precipitates as illness.

## ANNA : BREAST CANCER

What the mind has denied and blocked eventually writes itself on the body. And the diverse and complex symptoms — mental, emotional or physical — which arise as we go through life can often be used in their turn as direct pointers to those aspects of soul which are not being expressed.

Anna came to see us when she was having treatment for a second occurrence of breast cancer. She had first encountered the disease some fifteen years previously as an isolated nodule which had been removed in a "lumpectomy." As far as Anna was concerned, that was the end of it. She saw no greater meaning in the illness and tried hard to put it out of her mind as she plunged back into her busy career as teacher.

But then she discovered a lump in her other breast. Given the decade and a half that had elapsed, it seemed likely the recurrence was a completely new tumour, rather than a secondary metastases, spreading from the original site. And this time, Anna sat up and took notice. She realized that the cancer had always arisen when she had been under great personal and work-related stress; and she felt suspicious that this stress had compromised her immune system and that her decreased immunity might have something to do with her susceptibility to cancer. In any case, she wasn't willing to take any more chances and began to seek out ways to both reduce and cope more effectively with the stress in her life.

If she had been in any doubt, returning to her work environment after radiotherapy convinced her that she had to do something. She saw that her colleagues were all sick or burned out and realized that if she simply returned to work she could expect to be ill again very quickly. She knew that she could not drain her energy at work as she once had and hope to contend successfully with her illness.

None of her physicians, however, would pay more than lip service to these issues. Her surgeon said he'd done his job and that was the end of it. The oncologist who had treated her with radiation and chemotherapy hid behind a barrage of statistics to avoid further discussion. And her family doctor told her to put the whole thing behind her and get on with her life.

No doubt they all meant well. They just didn't see the need to explore issues they felt weren't relevant. To them, breast cancer was just a physical diagnosis. There was no greater issue than that. But Anna was not convinced.

Like so many of the people we see in our work, Anna was dissatisfied with the denial of her deeper issues. Who she was, why she worked where she did and why she submitted herself to so much stress seemed to her now real questions, questions she was now interested to ask.

## THE DENIAL MECHANISM

Anna loved teaching but hated the paperwork and red tape and the endless meetings that went with her job. Still, she was a people-pleaser who found it impossible to say no or to set boundaries. Consequently, she tended to take on more and more work until she had far more than she wanted. And it wasn't the kind of work she enjoyed. It took her further and further away from her first love which was to be with her students. She was always giving herself away.

I asked her if she ever did anything for herself. "No," she replied, "I would feel much too guilty."

"But what if you had only six months to live?" I posited. "What would you do?"

"I'd work," she replied. "I couldn't just walk away from the children and my commitments."

"What if you only had three months?" I pressed her.

"Ah, well, I suppose if I really knew that I only had three months, I might go to South America. I've always wanted to go there," she finally admitted.

"Aren't you leaving it a bit late to do something for yourself?" I enquired. "Leaving doing something you've always wanted to do till the last three months of your life."

"Yes, I suppose I am," she admitted. "But you know, the children really need me, and anyway, we've just put an additional wing on the house and we have a big mortgage to pay."

"What use is a house to you, or you to your students, if you are dead?" I asked rather bluntly.

Anna started to cry. "I know you're right," she murmured. "But I just can't think about it. It's too painful know that I might die. Better to keep working than to feel that."

## OWNING ONE'S LIFE AND OWNING ONE'S DEATH

Anna had touched the wound which drove her on. The need to please, the need to be needed, to keep busy, to be useful, were all manifestations of her denial of her own personhood — her own life and her own death. She worked as compulsively and as *selfless*ly as she did to deny her self, and so deny her mortality; to escape the fear of facing her own death: that is, facing her self.

Anna thought duty and debt kept her at work. But deep inside, she began to realize, she was afraid of herself. If she turned to "face" her own life, she must face her death, too. And this fear kept her from ever letting go.

Many of us would rather grasp at a straw than confront this intimate, profound and inevitable part of all our lives. So we often see little option but to submit our bodies to further and further insult in the vague hope of another few days of life.

But something was turning in Anna. Chemotherapy and radiotherapy, she knew, could offer only marginal benefits in her particular situation. And placing her trust in them might lead her inexorably to her grave. Moreover, she was beginning to intuit another way to heal.

## GETTING BEYOND "CAUSE"

The world is an infinitely complex place so just how or why a specific illness manifests is anybody's guess but Anna understood clearly that her cancer was calling her to take a look at herself. Perhaps if she chose to see her cancer as a wake up call, she might make some interesting discoveries. Already she was beginning to see that her habit of responsibility allowed her to live her life for others rather than allow her spirit its own expression; and that to live this life she had long had to deny her intuition and put aside her deepest feelings.

She had equated "being herself" with irresponsibility and had difficulty reconciling the two. As a result, there was a part of herself which was never allowed full expression. But now she faced a situation serious enough to challenge her assumptions and her priorities. Suddenly it was clear that her pride in her responsibility and rationality might be misplaced if these virtues invited her annihilation. Her illness was literally putting her life on the line and Anna knew something else was needed.

Such contradictions are a part of everyone's psyche. *Deep inside everyone who is ill, I believe, is a contradiction so crucial that it would seem that annihilation would accompany full expression of the soul.*

Anna's intuition was strong but she had never allowed herself to follow it. Her ego was attached to her image of herself as a woman dutiful in meeting her work and community obligations and paying her mortgage. To her mind, intuition threatened to annihilate her by tempting her to redefine her responsibilities.

## CATALYSTS

In the chemistry lab, a "catalyst" is a factor which is necessary for a reaction to proceed. In holistic medicine, a catalyst is that which allows the precipitation of illness in susceptible individuals.

Once an illness is present in a kind of suspended animation or "virtual reality," all it needs is a catalyst in order to precipitate or manifest. Because they are the proverbial "last straw," we often misinterpret these catalysts as the "cause" of the disease — especially when we wish to deny our illness's deeper roots.

In other words, in assessing the circumstances of an illness, we can pick any "cause" we like. If we believe in germs, we will look for germs. If we believe in nutrition, we will blame our diet. If we believe in toxic chemicals in the environment, we'll blame them. No doubt all of these are factors in many illnesses, but none are the cause of any particular illness. They are simply the triggers, or catalysts. (While Anna intuited that stress had caused her cancer, her physicians denied it. Joe might have blamed his smoking while the medical establishment fingered the streptococcus and I as a young doctor wondered about his sense of lonely isolation.)

## MOVING TOWARDS OUR OWN LIGHT

Whatever the "real" cause, it is certain that understanding illness as blocked spirit allows us to be creative and pro-active in our healing where otherwise we might despair. But it's not an intellectual thing. The route to change is through an intuitive understanding of the spiritual nature of the problem. As long as

Anna was preoccupied with worry about her statistical chances, she remained in despair. But once she embraced her intuition and saw that her illness might have meaning, there was a beacon of light in her darkness.

That light in the darkness signals the change in mind and spirit — the literal "enlightenment" — which is necessary for healing to occur. With that shift comes a relaxation of the tension which in turn releases huge resources of trapped energy. Everything is suddenly transformed.

Chapter 6

# REVERSAL

*Grace strikes us when we are in great pain and
restlessness. ... Sometimes at that moment a wave
of light breaks into the darkness, and it is as
though a voice were saying, 'You are accepted.'*

— Paul Tillich

Reversal of illness normally requires much the same
ingredients as did its precipitation. Falling ill and healing are
like two sides of a coin; and if we can turn the coin one way,
albeit unconsciously, then we should be able to turn it back.

But the unpalatable truth is that physical illness is not automatically reversed when we do everything right — change our
attitudes, pay attention to our constitutional weaknesses, meditate, exercise, take vitamins and supplements, consult different
healers, explore our illness's meanings — any more than an illness precipitates automatically when we do something unwise.
It would be nice if there was a formula we could follow which
would guarantee healing but unfortunately the body-mind-
spirit isn't that simple.

Once illness has arisen in us, it can take a number of different
courses. In some cases, healing is completely unconscious and our
pain or disease disappears as quickly and mysteriously as it arose.
Or, we may find a physician or practitioner who "fixes" our problem. In this case, we may attribute our healing to the skill of the
practitioner or to some prescribed medication. But sometimes illness becomes entrenched despite our efforts to rid ourselves of it
and we may despair.

## GRACE : UNPREDICTABLE HEALING

Symptoms sometimes disappear, as they appear, for no apparent reason; and spontaneous remissions of more serious diseases do happen. In fact, health practitioners soon learn that however determined we are to approach illness rationally, as often as not something irrational enters the fray, catalyzing healing and leaving us amazed. After all, since healing a particular ill is by definition something we haven't done before, its nature will always be unknown until it is experienced.

In other words, healing — like the rest of life — is inherently unpredictable: there is always something about it which defies explanation and prediction. Just as we may feel unlucky when illness arises, so we may feel lucky when it evaporates. Indeed, rapid improvements in our health can be so awesome they may seem a manifestation of "grace" — as though the universe has turned its radiance on us. And to expect — and welcome — the unexpected is probably the best we can do.

But the movement of grace that begins to heal us does not have to be a huge or breathtaking thing, although it may well be. Rather, it could be something completely ordinary, something almost imperceptible — unless we are watching for it.

## IRA : ACUTE BACK PAIN, DEPRESSION

Ira was a friend of mine, a generally healthy fellow in his late forties who felt he was quite well apart from occasional bouts of back pain. Over the years, we had often talked at length about the concepts of energy medicine. He had had little direct experience with it, however, until one day, quite without warning, his back went out as never before.

It was early evening when my phone rang. Ira was on the other end. His normally relaxed manner was replaced by tense urgency as he asked if I would come around to see him. He was obviously rather embarrassed and offered several apologies for bothering me at such an inconvenient time of day. Knowing Ira as I did, I felt certain he must be in fairly serious trouble to call me.

When I went round to his house, I found him lying prostrate on his bed in real agony, trying desperately to maintain his usual cool, but blanching with every movement. It was impossible not to notice that every time he shifted a fraction, his right leg shook uncontrollably. There was little doubt this was the same myoclonic activity I was familiar with from working with people in chronic pain, but here it was exhibiting itself in the throes of an acute incident — no doubt the body's innate healing ability responding to a physical insult.

It seemed an ideal opportunity to encourage Ira to consciously engage the healing power of his body, and I told him so, suggesting that he experiment with giving his body the freedom to move as it wanted and resisting the temptation to take drugs which might freeze the release of energy he was experiencing.

I knew that Ira was not keen on drugs in any case so, in spite of his discomfort, I found him fairly open to allowing his body a chance to heal itself. Still he was in intractable pain and had been for most of the day and was getting quite frightened by the whole ordeal — as was his wife, who was bearing the brunt of it all as caregiver, and who needed reassurance, too.

I thought some acupuncture might relieve enough of the pain to allow Ira to further encourage the energetic reaction he was experiencing. Body acupuncture proved tricky because he was in so much distress; so we moved to the ear, which I have found is remarkably relevant to acute back pain. Eventually, I found a point on his left ear which seemed appropriate and put a small press tack on it.

Ira immediately relaxed and, looking astonished, said his pain was half what it had been and he could feel heat rising up his back to envelop his head and left ear. He was more than willing to carry on with his exploration, so I left instructions on how he was to work with the myoclonus and left for home.

Ira called three days later to say he was beginning to get up and move around a bit. He said he had managed to avoid pain killers, using the shaking technique whenever necessary, several times a day as his body dictated. I hoped he was over the hill and thought he would continue to improve.

But it wasn't that easy. Despite his faithful daily shaking, Ira's recovery was halting. There seemed to be a missing factor, some block or lack. Although he was able to get up, he continued to be very fatigued and felt generally unwell, with an upset stomach and intermittent back pain. And as time wore on, he was gradually sinking into fear and depression, wondering why he was not getting better.

In his despair, Ira started to think there might be something seriously wrong. He consulted his regular physician, who suggested the problem was probably due to a lingering infection and initiated a series of blood and urine tests, and backed them up with low back and kidney x-rays. The next thing he knew, Ira was taking antibiotics for a presumed urinary tract infection and was told he might have a kidney stone.

Next, the side effects of the antibiotics kicked in, interfering with his appetite and giving him diarrhoea, leaving him even more alarmed at what was happening to his body. He knew he was taking the antibiotics for dubious reasons, but didn't know what else to do, and fear was in control. I could see that despite his knowledge of energy medicine, Ira was falling into the same traps anyone might. It seems knowledge cannot help us avoid whatever lessons are out there for us. We have to live our lives and our experience directly to understand.

## A WALK IN THE GARDEN

After another couple of weeks mostly spent lying in bed wondering why he was not improving, Ira got fed up with himself and decided that no matter how terrible he felt, he absolutely had to get out. He'd been lying around for too long, he thought; maybe he should sit in the sun for a while, or walk in his garden.

But then a funny thing happened. When after much pain and physical negotiation he got himself outside, Ira felt how good it was to be in the fresh air after being cooped up for so long, and almost immediately noticed that he felt a little better. He even felt like pulling the odd weed, particularly as his garden was looking a little the worse for six weeks of neglect. Soon he was feeling better still, and before he knew it he'd spent half an hour enjoying the dirt under his hands. So the next day he thought he would go out again, and again the next. Soon he seemed to "forget" his back pain, his fatigue, and his general unwellness and was back to his old self, having learned the lesson of the unpredictable. I spoke to him about the whole experience sometime later and there was no doubt in his mind that his garden had cured what all the medicines in the world were powerless to affect. But it was not a rational event. He had gone out into the garden on the strength of an inner impulse generated from anger.

Unfortunately, we cannot command the irrational to present itself. All we can do is make sure we have done everything possible to move in the direction of wellness and then wait for a catalyst. The natural unpredictability of life will present any number of non-rational situations. We have only to be able to acknowledge and welcome the catalyst when it arrives.

## KAREN : RHEUMATOID ARTHRITIS

The place of the unpredictable in healing illness is always fascinating. We ponder and rationalize until we think we have everything figured out but there is always another factor needed for healing to occur, and that other factor is often irrational.

Karen was a 55-year-old woman who came to our clinic after struggling with rheumatoid arthritis for seven years. The illness had come on shortly after her husband died of cancer. Prior to that, she had considered herself quite healthy, and the tragic context of the illness's advent seemed eerily relevant.

Karen had been taking anti-inflammatory agents (NSAIDS), prednisone and, more recently, methotrexate to help her function. She feared the potential side-effects of these drugs, particularly methotrexate which she knew could cause liver damage. So while methotrexate appeared to control her symptoms, the longer she took it the more desperately worried she became. Finally, she realized she had to look for more profound healing so that she could get off the medication she felt was so dangerous.

Karen jumped into her exploratory work with us with great enthusiasm. She was extremely dynamic during bodywork sessions and on the third day began myoclonic activity which continued for several hours. While she could stop it consciously if she chose, the moment she relaxed it would start up again. In the end, Karen shook intermittently for several days, her symptoms improving hour by hour as the stagnant energy in her body began to shift and move. She was ecstatic at her improvement, and keen to keep going, like a marathon athlete going the extra mile. Toward the end of ten days she was virtually pain-free.

Karen felt she was well on her way to a cure, but we cautioned her. Her methotrexate was administered weekly by injection, and her last dose was just before she arrived. Only time would tell if her remission would last. We tried to warn Karen not to be disappointed if her symptoms returned but to remember to work with them rather than against them, in the way she had learned. She had of course made a very encouraging start as it showed her — and us — what was possible.

During the initial phases of the exploratory process, we will often get this sort of glimpse of the future. Indeed, but for this glimpse it's doubtful many would persist on the rough and rocky road, full of pitfalls and heartaches, which make up so many healing journeys — it's sometimes all we have to hold onto when the journey gets tough.

Such was the case for Karen, who had two blissful weeks before an altercation with her mother precipitated a return of her symptoms. Within moments, she could feel the tension returning to her body and, a few short hours later, her joints began to stiffen and swell up.

Karen refused to be disheartened, however, convinced from her initial experience that she could get back on track. She returned with high hopes — and this time without her methotrexate. But despite her best efforts, Karen did not improve. Instead, she got worse and by the end of the program was so stiff she could hardly walk. Understandably depressed, she tried dietary changes, herbal remedies and a water fast. In the end nothing worked, and Karen was forced to return to her medication for some relief.

This disappointment forced Karen to dig deeper into her pain, deeper than she had ever been willing to go before. In total despair, she began to reckon with the possibility that her illness might never leave her. It was the one thing, she told us, she had never allowed herself to think.

But by allowing such feelings, she made an important connection: she realized such despair was strangely familiar and without much trouble traced the feeling to the time when her husband had died a few years previously. When he died, she felt that a light had gone out in her life; and she recalled consciously suppressing an anguished and frightening hopelessness shortly before her illness had begun.

When we encouraged her to feel back through these feelings, she began to understand that at some level she had resolved never to experience them again. Her subconscious seemed to think the solution was fairly simple: if love meant risking such terrible loss, she must never allow herself to feel deeply for anyone again. At that moment, it seemed that a primal instruction had been broadcast throughout the body-mind: "Do something (short of dying) to absolutely ensure I will not have to face a love relationship again!" There, Karen intuited, was the elusive meaning behind her symptoms.

After that insight, Karen changed. Gone were the naïve expectations of miracle cures, the belief in a magic bullet. In their place was a deep willingness to face herself and her disease. She was back on a slightly reduced dose of methotrexate, her joints were mildly inflamed, but she was mobile — and determined.

## THE NATURE OF EXPECTATION

Now just at this moment there was a man, John, visiting our centre who had discovered the gift of healing in his hands. He wasn't really sure how it worked but it was there. One day volunteered to put his hands on Karen's sore knees.

It was nothing extraordinary, just an unplanned encounter. But in that moment, Karen felt touched by grace. An unexpected event had entered her life. Afterward, she felt energized, stronger, as well as more centred and calm, as if something in her had shifted. Her joints began to settle once again.

After a long preparation and an encounter with profound despair, it seemed Karen had discovered her catalyst. She had done everything she could to heal, without much lasting success, and had moved beyond naïve hope to acceptance. She was eating wisely, had cut down on her drugs, and had explored her illness's meaning in her life. There was little else she could do but trust that if healing was to happen, the universe would take care of the details. She was open to anything — the new, the strange and the unexpected — and it was then that grace entered her life.

Life is so inherently unpredictable, if we just trust that healing could happen, are open to the unusual and willing to learn from others, it seems there is no limit to what can occur. I talked to Karen several months after she left us. Her joints had not flared up in that time, and she had halved her dose of methotrexate. The great mystery of the unpredictable remains as tantalizing as ever.

Part III

WOUNDS

Chapter 7

# BOUNDARIES & THE VOID

*Repressing emotions can only be causative of disease.*
*A common ingredient in the healing practices of native*
*cultures is catharsis, complete release of emotion.*

— Candace Pert

In life, where we must balance the apparently conflicting demands of separateness and connectedness, our boundaries demarcate our separateness. As infants, we have no boundaries to speak of and generally behave as if the world were a part of our self and ourself a part of the world. Later, our experiences of helplessness and vulnerability prompt us to begin to establish boundaries which give us a sense of identity and protectedness. And because our Western culture tends to value separateness over connectedness, understanding boundaries as essential to individualism, much of our growing up involves defining and defending these boundaries as a way of stating who we are and of understanding our place in the universe. Thus begins our separation from all around us.

## HEALING AND PERSONAL BOUNDARIES

The firmness and location of personal boundaries depend on each person's experience. Our physical boundaries are often assumed to be projected out a short way beyond our bodies. But each of us has further, wider spheres — such as family, property, profession, race and nationality — and each of these functions to provide a sense of security, order and identity in an otherwise uncertain world. We hold them dear because they appear to protect and define us.

When pain or illness steps into our carefully constructed separateness and demands to be heard, it threatens to destroy our self-sufficiency, our ego and everything it stands for. It is no wonder, then, that we are so alarmed by it. But as well as breaching our boundaries, pain can itself act as a boundary, sealing off territory within ourselves which we adamantly refuse to explore. Strange as it may seem, pain — or any other chronic symptom — can become the toughest of barriers to self-knowledge; and though we spend so much energy trying to get rid of it, in order to heal we must somehow embrace our pain.

The true task of the healer, then, is not to relieve symptoms, as the Hippocratic oath would suggest, but to facilitate and encourage the process already set in motion by helping individuals to explore their illnesses. It is during the process of integration — which constitutes a large part of the healing journey — that our most personal boundaries are breached and our soul transcends the ego-bounded self, the "I."

The threat to the ego involved in confronting its boundaries is usually perceived as very great, and the guide must persuade the seeker to cross or dissolve boundaries he or she doesn't particularly want to cross — or even know about. This places the healer in a most difficult position. How can she or he work with people so that their egos won't be offended?

VIOLENCE AGAINST THE SELF: THE SOUL SPEAKS FIERCELY

Surprisingly, the answer is partly through a thorough exploration of the issue of violence. As civilized beings, we don't often acknowledge our capacity for violence, preferring to project it onto others then fearfully rejecting them so we don't have to confront the issue. But by creating illness or addiction, by engineering an accident, or by indulging in other self-destructive behaviours, our soul serves notice that it is not averse to using violence as a means of getting our attention.

We have little choice, then, but to address the violence within us; and, through an honest exploration, come to understand what our soul is trying to achieve. The issue is central to the healing journey and we cannot avoid it if we wish to heal.

## RECLAIMING VIOLENT ENERGIES

Though healing is usually seen as a process of care and nurture, a significant part of it also involves becoming aware of our shadow and reclaiming our violent energies. While illness might seem a noble solution to the problem of repressed violence — better to injure the self than others, the ego might rationalize — it is ultimately a doomed strategy.

Illness is after all not a terrific way to solve the problem of living; and it's unfortunate that so many of us seem to choose it, albeit unconsciously, as a focus for and expression of our lives. Far better, I think, to become aware of our shadow energies, and learn to channel and gradually integrate that energy into ourselves, making it available for more life-affirming uses and defusing its destructive potential.

## ROBERT : ANGER AND ENERGETIC IMBALANCE

I'll never forget Robert, a 32-year-old mechanic. Five years earlier, the hydraulic lift supporting a car he was working on had failed. He was nearly crushed to death when the car came down on top of him but managed to hold off the front end long enough for his friends to help him. He survived the accident but went on to develop massive pain in his neck, shoulders and upper back, and incapacitating headaches. Over the years, he had tried every conceivable therapy to no avail and had become thoroughly enraged with the medical profession.

Robert's anger was so strong it was palpable. I could feel it before he even opened his mouth. As a result, our first conversation was not easy. He was reluctant to tell me anything and was almost monosyllabic in his replies to my questions. No doubt from his point-of-view I was just another in a long line of doctors who had so far done nothing for him. But with perseverance I managed to get some of his history. Robert was born with a cleft palate and had spent a lot of time in hospital as a young child having corrective surgery. Otherwise, his upbringing had been fairly straightforward and he had had no other serious medical problems until his recent injury. I wondered in passing whether his early hospitalizations could have contributed subconsciously to his present anger.

I admit I found it difficult to like Robert. He seemed a raging cauldron ready to explode at any moment. He made absolutely no effort to be friendly yet I knew he must desperately need his pain to be validated. Had I been less aware of the energetics of anger, I might have declined to continue the relationship but something told me to stick it out.

When we began working together, I noticed that while above his neck the skin was hot to the touch below the neck it was noticeably cold. His hands and feet were almost icy. And though Robert put a lot of effort into his sessions, no matter what we tried there never seemed to be any movement of energy sufficient to shift the markedly abnormal hot/cold distribution.

Eventually, Robert and I built a working relationship which had at least some elements of the trust so necessary for significant progress; and he began to realize the depth of his rage and that, finally, he was in a context safe enough to explore it.

One day, rather unexpectedly, Robert entered the void. Up to that point, he had been deep breathing with great gusto but without much in the way of results. On this particular day, however, he had different look on his face; there was a fire in his eye which I didn't pay much attention to at the time but which in retrospect I realized had signalled a shift in his intention.

Perhaps he had decided to trust me, I don't know, but within minutes of taking a couple of deep breaths he catapulted into the void and his face turned a deep puce colour. Then, without warning, his hands suddenly shot up, encircled my neck and began to squeeze until I had difficulty breathing. I fell back on the floor and relaxed. I had no idea what was going to happen next but for a moment I honestly wondered whether it was to be my last day on the planet.

After an interminable ten or fifteen seconds, Robert let out a howl of rage, let me go, and sat down crying from deep in his belly. His body shook as paroxysms of rage and grief began to pour from him. For about twenty minutes his shoulders shuddered violently, his hands alternately trembling and pounding the ground. After it was over, he lay down where he was and fell asleep, deeply relaxed for perhaps the first time in years. I touched his hands and noticed they were warm.

Once the door to the void had been opened, it was simply a matter of going back several times until a permanent shift occurred in Robert's energetic structure. At the same time, although his rage at the medical profession remained, he warmed to me as an individual; and in spite of my experience, I no longer felt any fear around him. We had been to the brink together and survived. The fear of what he might do — his fear and mine — had not been realized. And by the time Robert left us, his headaches were much reduced and his hands and feet much warmer.

No doubt Robert's very early experiences in hospitals had seemed inexcusable violations of his boundaries which he had been powerless to protest or prevent. Later, when his injuries put him "at the mercy" of physicians again and they had been unable to help him, his anger, put away since childhood, had resurfaced. As a physician myself, I represented the original and continuing source of his rage. No wonder it had been so difficult for me to connect with him. Though his anger was against what I represented, not me personally, I felt it personally and was not able, at least initially, to make the distinction.

It has taken many years for me to understand this encounter — and others like it — and even now I still have great difficulty with it. It seems Robert's experience of boundary violation as a small child left him in the difficult position of needing to violate my boundaries in order to begin to heal. I've no doubt it took a monumental leap of trust for him to admit those feelings in my presence; and when I was able to look at the whole experience from that perspective, I felt almost honoured by such trust.

The truth is, many people with chronic pain or illness see the physician as an enemy to be feared, rather than the helper he or she is meant to be. Like injured animals, such people will sometimes bite the hand which is offered to help them.

## TOUGH LOVE

It might seem that if patients ask for the assistance of a therapist, they must want the changes necessary for healing, but this is rarely so. In most cases, we assume that personal boundaries will remain sacred. When the awful truth dawns on us that real change is required, we may turn and vent our rage on the healer rather than face the violence in ourselves.

The transcendence of ego boundaries demanded by the soul is a violent process and the buried energies which force the opening are often related to repressed rage and other difficult emotions, or to sexual issues, the expression none of which is condoned by society. A confident therapist must embody the principles of "tough love" — a phrase coined by people who work with recalcitrant teenagers — to avoid sympathetic collusion with an ego bent on avoidance of pain. In practice, this demands the therapist maintain a detached calmness in the presence of any difficult energies which might emerge from the void.

## BODYWORK

The issue of boundaries and their dissolution or confrontation has even greater import when it comes to "hands-on" work, as the challenge for the hands-on therapist is to help us explore our symptoms experientially by exposing the artificial boundary between our perceived self and the pain of our illness.

In hands-on work, the point of physical contact between therapist and client is the action point, the point where energy is exchanged and boundaries are felt and contested. If there are going to be difficulties in healing, they will occur at this point, for it is here that the healing relationship faces its biggest test. As the patient faces his pain and the therapist her potentially hostile patient, there can be a loss of trust on either one or both sides and the therapeutic relationship may well founder just when something is about to happen.

There is a fine edge between too little and too much, a place between pain and no pain, between what is acceptable and what is unacceptable. Too much pressure will result in a sense of violation and panicked resistance or anger; too little results in no movement and no healing. The competent bodyworker is neither violent nor non-violent, but enters the healing space — the void — at the contact point and, in effect, hangs there between the two, as though both violent and non-violent and yet beyond them both.

It was when we entered that space with Robert that his anger erupted. The experience of being on the edge of his pain no doubt triggered all the rage which was simmering just below the surface. Of course, a release of anger — since it represents a movement of energy — is not a problem if it is owned by the client and understood as impersonal by the therapist, though as we have mentioned, such an eruption can be so terrifying that both instinctively back off and resolve to avoid the same experience in the future. Really major difficulties arise when patients absolutely refuse to own their pain and take offence at any "hands-on" practices which result in the slightest discomfort, blaming the therapist for "causing" it. In this situation, the movement of healing energy is arrested until the question of who caused what has been clearly understood. If the client absolutely cannot own his or her anger, then trust is destroyed and healing will be deferred to another day.

I am reminded of one very hostile woman who refused all hands-on therapy. In the end, the only thing she would accept was some cupping — an ancient technique in which suction cups are put on the skin to promote blood flow to painful areas. We carefully explained the procedure to her and told her to expect some suction marks on her skin which would settle in a few days. While she found the procedure very acceptable at the time, she later had photographs taken of the marks and tried to use them as evidence of abuse in her litigation. Such are the difficulties when rage is projected and violence disowned.

One way or another, all people who come for help have some irreconcilable conflict like Robert's, the dynamics of which are unique to the individual, and difficult energies of one kind or another are present in everyone. Consequently, if we try to take the easy road — never pressing boundaries, avoiding conflict, or projecting our rage onto others, then we betray ourselves and will never cross the threshold into the void to find healing.

Unfortunately, crossing that threshold can be so frightening and the energies encountered so terrifying that patients and practitioners alike often flee the situation rather than face it. Few people are prepared to face the dynamic of uncontrolled emotional release and shy away when it happens. The guardian beast of the underworld can be pretty scary.

# Chapter 8

# CHILDHOOD TERRORS

*Nothing can be bought to an end in the unconscious;*
*nothing is past or forgotten*

— Sigmund Freud

We each seem to retain something of the child we once were within us. This child carries our hopes and fears and some of our more primal feelings. I have come to believe that this child controls far more than we realize, and is the motivator of many of our adult behaviours.

Childhood is a time when we are relatively helpless, and dependent on others for nearly everything. During this period, we learn about the world through the filter of our particular society's belief system; we learn what our elders consider right and wrong; are perhaps indoctrinated in the beliefs of a particular religious tradition; go to school; and are involved in adult/child power struggles and projections.

Our experiences as a child largely determine who we are and who we will become. If our parents are emotionally distant, we may become emotionally distant, or conversely, exceptionally needy. If we are physically abused, we may become abusive adults. If a parent is absent, we may have difficulty with our self-image. If one or other of our parents are alcoholic, we may feel tormented by unspecific guilt and become overachievers, and/or develop a similar addiction. In fact, though teenagers try their best to distinguish themselves from their parents, it is remarkable how often their rebellions actually create the similarity they are trying to avoid.

While the average adult can control or mask unresolved childhood traumas, as we reach old age these mechanisms can weaken, allowing the hurt and fearful child to reappear. I believe this is why we so often see older people regressing to childhood behaviours and behaving irrationally.

It makes sense then to try to come to terms with these fears at a time of life where we have the energy and the will to integrate our various contradictory feelings. Some people do this quite spontaneously, but many never do, and for others the integration gets delayed until illness forces the individual to confront the issues. Under such circumstances, illness may motivate us to seek the deeper understanding needed to integrate the feelings of the frightened child; indeed, if we would heed the urgings of the inner child, symptoms which seem inexplicable might be more easily understood.

When I was small, I remember being told that children should be seen and not heard. It seems this is a common admonition. Now I see patients who look like adults but sound like children trying to express themselves. Sometimes I wonder if that child within, who was told to be quiet, is still trying to find a way to be heard. In any case, and for whatever reason, I have seen many people benefit from the opportunity to integrate some of the buried feelings from those earlier years.

## MARGARET : PARANOIA

I will never forget an old patient of mine who returned to see me after several years. Margaret had originally come for treatment for a stiff neck and headaches. I had had to treat her for some months before the condition finally resolved and during that time we had established a friendly and trusting relationship. She was of the old school, a product of a fairly rigid Victorian upbringing, but with a little effort I could see beyond the stiff upper lip and propriety to a gentle — and frightened — little girl inside still waiting to express herself. When Margaret and I eventually parted, her shell had softened a bit, her stiff neck had gone and we had become friends.

After so long, I was surprised to hear from members of her family who felt that she was becoming paranoid. In particular, it seemed she complained of being followed, and insisted that the neighbour across the street was trying to get into the house during the night and harm her. Her family quite naturally thought that Margaret, now seventy-five, was beginning to lose her marbles. But the situation was serious enough that if things did not improve, she could end up in a home for the mentally infirm.

Not knowing what else to suggest, Margaret's physician had prescribed anti-psychotic medication to control her aberrant behaviour, and the family, at their wits' ends, was ready to submit her to the drugs. Margaret, however, was by no means ready to take them. She had been the drug route many years previously for her chronic headaches, and had found it unhelpful.

Another difficulty was that she didn't trust anyone. Her paranoia encompassed nearly all her relationships, including her family doctor. She had also refused to see a psychiatrist or any other health professional, convinced they would dope her and put her in a home. She might have been right.

For some reason, she was willing to see me. We talked at some length. After the usual formalities, we got down to the nitty gritty and I asked her what was really going on. She was very matter-of-fact, as was her wont, and told me that a number of recent events had come together to precipitate her crisis. Most of these events involved loss. Her brother had died; her favourite niece was getting married and moving to another part of town; and her own marriage had dissolved.

"My brother and I were extremely close," she said, bursting into tears. "I don't know what I am going to do without him. I always thought I would be the one to go first."

Her grief was intense.

"And my niece is planning to move. I don't want her to leave. ... She's been so good to me all these years, and now I won't be able to see her. I don't drive any more because of my eyes, so I can't just get in my car to go over to her new place. It's all very difficult. And of course it hasn't been easy since my husband left ... not that we were getting on very well but I was so used to his being around, the place feels empty without him."

Nothing so far had indicated anything more than situational stress. It all seemed very reasonable.

"Everything you've mentioned seems perfectly understandable," I told her gently. "But your family tells me you've been seeing things. For example, what about this person who keeps coming into the house at night?" I pressed her a little to try to probe the difficult area.

"Oh, our neighbour you mean." She stiffened a little at the thought. "Yes, I keep thinking he's coming into the house at night. I can hear him walking around the house sometimes. And then there is the matter of the squeaking in the corner cabinet in the bedroom which makes me think he's in there too. Nobody believes me you know, but I know he is there."

There it was: from reasonable grief we had tipped into irrational paranoia. I wondered how to approach the issue. In order to earn her trust, I knew I had to validate her experience, even though I didn't believe her. I also knew that trying to sort this sort of thing out rationally is completely futile, because feeling is at the root of it. The feeling was real, but where did it come from? I spent some time trying to link it to her grief but although she was clearly stricken by the loss of her family, her sadness was entirely understandable. The real problem lay elsewhere.

I decided to see if I could get anywhere by exploring the feeling itself. Perhaps by entering the feeling, we could find out what it was trying to express.

I asked her to repeat after me. " 'There's someone in the house ... there's someone in the house.' What do you feel in your body? What comes next?" She repeated the phrase several times. I encouraged her to explore what happened next. It didn't take long. "Oh ... that's the smell I get when he's in the house."

"What smell? What's it like?" I asked.

"I don't know," she said, "but it's a bit like stale smoke from my husband's pipe."

"Okay, let's go again. There's someone in the house. There's someone in the house. ... There's a funny smell, a funny smell, a funny smell. ... What's next?"

"There's a squeaking in the cupboard. I know someone's in there. There's noises coming from the cabinet." She started to get frightened.

"Okay, let's go to the cupboard and see what's in there."

Margaret's eyes were closed and she breathed a little faster as she entered the void. Her inner experience was becoming increasingly real to her as we spoke. In her mind's eye, Margaret went to the cabinet door, opened it and looked around inside. I was reminded of the little cupboard in the Narnia stories which opened one side into the room, and the other side into another world altogether. In a way, I expected something similar to happen, but on this particular day it was not to be so. All Margaret found in the cupboard amongst the clothes was a wall of blackness and fear.

On a subsequent day, Margaret again entered the void and headed for the cupboard.

"There's someone in the house, there's someone in the house," Margaret repeated as she crossed the threshold into the void. "I'm alone, I'm alone. There's a funny smell, and the cupboard is squeaking."

I had wondered whether the feelings of aloneness and panic were old, old feelings re-asserting themselves through the weakened defences of old age. And as she spoke I noticed that her voice was becoming increasingly childlike. Suddenly I understood that it really was a child talking. Perhaps here, I thought, was the frightened child finally making herself heard. I was not to be disappointed.

"Margaret," I said gently, "your voice sounds to me like you are quite a small child. Can you remember the room you were in when you were very small. If you can, I want you to go back to a time when you were that little child, and remember the room you slept in. Can you do that?" I coaxed her.

"Oh yes ... I can see it now." Her voice became animated. "The room is very dark, and I am all alone. There's no-one in the house. There's a cupboard in the corner of the room which squeaks. I imagine there are all kinds of monsters in that cupboard, so I hide under my blanket and never look out. I am absolutely terrified."

Margaret began to cry as she went over the events of so long ago; and as the story emerged, she spoke through her tears, and her body began to shake with the familiar myoclonus indicative of the movement of energy in the void. I knew we were onto something. Here was a little girl, sitting in her room in the dark, feeling alone and frightened, and hearing the squeak of the cupboard, in exactly the same way the elder Margaret was. The parallel was so striking that the conclusion was inescapable.

Far from developing a psychosis, or Alzheimer's disease, Margaret was simply re-experiencing a very frightening childhood situation. No doubt during her life, her adult coping skills were more than sufficient to conceal her inner terror — from others and in particular from herself. As her defences weakened with old age, the feelings of terror from childhood had re-emerged and come to the fore.

## ENERGY IMPRINTS : THE BODY'S MEMORIES

Margaret's story is far from unique. My experience suggests that many symptoms have their origin in some unresolved trauma long since buried. Given the right circumstance, those who have been injured in an accident will return to the scene and re-enact the moment, and others will experience some long-forgotten moment and finally understand its meaning. Either way, trauma can leave an impression on the body-mind, which will over time become energy imprints in the body's electromagnetic field.

Practitioners' experiences with energy imprints seem remarkably consistent. Craniosacral therapy talks of "energy cysts," Scientology talks of "engrams," and Traditional Chinese Medicine talks of "Qi and Blood stagnation." It seems that intense experience — whether physical or emotional, injury or accident — forms an imprint and that imprint will influence our behaviour in a way which reflects the original experience. Not surprisingly, clearing the body of such a charge is key to restoring the body and mind to health; and this clearing is accomplished somewhat paradoxically by re-entering the memory in an altered state of consciousness and re-experiencing the feelings buried there with it until the charge on them is reduced to a tolerable level.

But clearing the charge does not mean getting rid of the memory itself. To attempt to do so amounts to an intensified suppression which works temporarily at best, as suppression is ultimately what lies behind the emergence of symptoms.

Margaret entered the void on several other occasions and over time succeeded in reducing the charge on her childhood abandonment. She began to take an interest in her life again and seemed less controlled by her fears. She even was able to go to her niece's wedding. Her case really brought home to me the value of respecting individual experience, and fully trusting that it is valid, even though it may seem irrational. Anything less, in this case, would have taken Margaret down the slippery slope of pharmaceuticals, into a life of drug dependence from which she might never have emerged.

Unfortunately, as a society we make this tragic mistake time and time again. Rather than investigating our accumulated traumas, we try to diagnose the symptoms away, labelling instead of exploring them, or suppressing them with drugs. And in fact we cannot blame medicine entirely, because ultimately we make the choice ourselves. In my experience, few people are really prepared to explore their symptoms. Most will only consider it when there is no other option available. Until then, they will still be looking for an easy way out.

"I'll do anything except that," is a phrase I often hear when clients consider their options in exploring their symptoms. It's clear to me now that the "that" — whatever it is — is quite likely to be exactly the place they need to go.

Chapter 9

# THE SEXUAL WOUND

*Here everything is distorted and disowned,*
*although it is from this deepest*
*of all events that we come forth,*
*and have ourselves the centre of our ecstasies in it.*

— Rainer Maria Rilke

*T*here is one issue which I believe fragments the soul more than anything else and makes us feel less than whole. The shaming of our sexuality leads to feelings of anxiety and self-loathing, produces self-destructive behaviour, and may in the long run lead to illness. One way or another it affects everyone and so is of prime concern in the healing journey. But open discussion of sexual issues in the therapeutic milieu is often difficult — so difficult that the subject is usually avoided altogether.

It is my view that soul fragmentation and the shaming of our sexuality are reflections of the mind/body split to which I have previously alluded. The Cartesian view continually denies the validity of the body's experience and emphasizes the superiority of the intellect with the result that some of us live almost entirely in our heads and forget how to listen to our bodies. And while we can function that way in the rational world, we tend to run into trouble when it comes to matters of the heart. Tending to separate rather than connect, the intellect is a notoriously unreliable guide to love relationships.

## THE SEXUAL WOUND

It is my impression from experiential exploration and bodywork sessions with clients over the years that the way we experience our sexual energy is of prime importance to our health. A blockage in the flow of that energy is often intimately related to the genesis of illness.

Many people, in fact, seem to experience their sexuality as split off from the wholeness of their being, operating as an almost autonomous function. Such isolated sexual feeling, having no natural context, has to be forcibly restrained in order that we may function in the world. This wholesale repression tends to lump it in with other suppressed emotions. When control is weakened for whatever reason and unintegrated sexuality emerges confusedly allied with feelings of anger and fear and guilt, it can be frightening.

The shaming of our sexuality and the sexual wound which results are the subject of *The Incest Taboo*, by psychologist Robert Stein. According to Stein, the incest taboo, which is common to most human societies, functions to preclude sexual relationship where there is the closest spiritual relationship — such as between brother and sister, or child and parent — and those who transgress it generally face very severe societal condemnation. It is unlikely, however, that such taboos have ever been intended to denigrate sexuality itself but rather to channel it for the good of the society as a whole. Indeed many traditional societies developed coming-of-age rituals precisely to help youths learn life-enhancing ways of integrating their developing sexuality.

In the modern Western world, however, children very often have to figure out the meaning of sexuality on their own in a society blaring its unease, repressed violence and immaturity from every billboard and magazine advertisement. Consequently, for many young people, sexuality is shrouded in shame and secrecy; and learning about sex means picking up attitudes and misinformation from peers, films and magazines.

In the absence of mentoring or friendly guidance from a sympathetic adult, I and most of my peers were made to feel that we were wrong somehow, fundamentally bad or distorted in some way. As children, most of us simply did not have the ability to deal creatively with our emerging sexual feelings so we had little option but to solve the problem by suppression, especially as we saw few adults who didn't carry the same wound.

The shaming of one's sexuality can lead to a profound sense of inadequacy, low self-esteem and a tragic alienation of sexuality from feeling. Naturally, this love/sex split profoundly affects intimate relationships in those of us who come to adulthood with the issue unresolved. Because the incest taboo teaches us to suppress sexual feelings with the people we are closest to, as adults we may find difficulty bringing love and sexuality together.

Obviously there are degrees of wounding and many people manage to find a way through these difficulties. But for those of us with a significant split, the attempt to bring love and sexuality together can produce a sense of impending doom, as we tread close to the taboo. In order to circumvent such terror, we learn to suppress our sexuality in love relationships and to suppress our feelings in sexual relationships.

The result is a deep distrust of our bodies and our sexuality, and a feeling of shame which permeates and denigrates our intimate relationships. A man, for example, may find he has lost a friendship the moment a relationship becomes sexual; or loses a wonderful lover once a commitment is made. A woman may find she cannot sustain a meaningful relationship and is constantly on the move; or feels sexually aroused only with an abusive partner. The varieties of torment are endless but one thing is fairly sure: few people escape the wound altogether.

IAN : CHRONIC FATIGUE AND BACK PAIN

Ian was a 43-year-old man who came to me for help during a bout of acute anxiety and emotional turmoil. A former construction worker, he had been in a series of accidents which left him unable to carry on with the heavy physical demands of his job. The accidents were not particularly serious but they had left him chronically fatigued and in persistent pain.

Ian had first put his back out lifting a heavy beam; and was just recovering from that when he was sideswiped by a careless driver. Then, finally back at work, he tripped and hit his chest on a heavy oak chest. He was left with intermittent headaches and a lot of upper back and shoulder pain, and two years after this series of accidents, had still not recovered his health. Ian decided it was time to make some major changes in his life.

He had been diagnosed with fibromyalgia and chronic fatigue, and was living on a long-term disability pension. Realizing that he wanted to do something more with his life, he decided to fulfil a lifelong ambition to study art and enrolled in a four-year program at a local art school.

There was little doubt the change was good for him. He began to enjoy life again and feel better about himself. Pretty soon, he fell in love. Ian had been in relationships before but had never managed anything long-term. This time, however, things looked different. Ian and Leslie spent a lot of time together, and soon began to share their thoughts and feelings with each other; and their physical relationship was exciting and fulfilling. Life seemed very good indeed and, for the first time, Ian found he was beginning to feel secure with a woman. Finally, he thought, things were going his way.

But then one day it all came to an end. First Leslie didn't return a phone call. Then she began avoiding him. If he ran into her at a party, she would be cordial but not intimate. Eventually she refused to talk to him at all, or even acknowledge him, acting as though he wasn't present. The closeness and security he so desperately wanted was gone. In its place was coldness and distance.

He tried to communicate his pain but got nowhere: Leslie seemed to have gone into a shell. Ian began to fall apart. He couldn't focus on his art, his stomach was upset, his appetite was gone and he began to lose weight. If people spoke to him, he often wouldn't hear. He was suffering the torments of a lovesick teenager but at midlife it was more than he bargained for.

Ian had stumbled upon the sexual wound which he'd been able to keep buried for many years. Though he could understand rejection intellectually, he was shattered. He felt that just as he had finally been able to open his heart to a woman, he was being betrayed. Though he felt that at his age he should be able to handle it, the pain he was feeling was intense and omnipresent. It spoke to something deeper.

## A COMMON DILEMMA

Ian's experience is not unique. Indeed, it is so common it seems to speak to a universal phenomenon. Ian could have a sexual relationship with a woman as long as she didn't get too close. He could be friends with a woman as long as he didn't have sex with her. But the moment he tried to bring the two together, the relationship was somehow destroyed. Just when he was getting close to what he wanted, he lost it.

Ian was very keen to do some bodywork to explore the problem. He had investigated every other avenue at his disposal to come to terms with his feelings and he knew he was stuck. He had talked to his counsellor, and his physician, had tried to question the feeling through meditation, but there seemed to be an impenetrable wall beyond which he could not go. We decided to probe that wall using acupuncture and breathing to enter the void.

With the insertion of the first needle Ian's right hand began to tremble and shake. Soon he was sighing; then he began to cry and to talk through his tears.

"Why did you do this? Why? Why?" he railed. "I loved you. I shared myself with you. I made it so safe for you to be who you are. Why did you do this to me?" Ian started with the poor-me approach. Then he began to get angry.

"I could just shake you!" His fists clenched up. "I could shake you till you break apart. Why won't you listen to me? Why won't you answer my calls? We could sort this out if you would just listen." His voice got louder.

Then he began to pound his fists on the mat. "Damn you anyway. Damn you! damn you! damn you!" Each damn brought a tightly clenched fist down on the mat with a vengeance. Ian was beginning to shake all over like leaf.

I sensed the feelings Ian had were very old, probably from his childhood, so I tossed it out to him. "Stay with it Ian," I encouraged him. "Keep the deep breathing rhythm. Feel the energy running through you. This feeling is very old. It's been there for a long time. Let it speak to you."

"Never like this," he replied.

"Are you sure?" I queried. "Stay with it, let it speak to you."

Ian kept shaking from his toes to the tip of his head.

"Oh! ...... " he suddenly announced. "I *have* had this feeling before — probably fifteen years ago. You know I had totally forgotten about her. I haven't thought about Celia in years. We had been together for a year when she suddenly left." He got more angry.

"Women are all the same. They give you the big come on then they dump you. I hate them all," he screamed at the top of his lungs. Ian's hands were shaking, his teeth were chattering, and his body was literally vibrating off the mat.

I felt we were getting close, but we were still not there.

"Aaagh!" Ian shouted in total exasperation, and then he seemed to relax somewhat. When he had settled a bit more he began to explain, "You know, you're right. I have had this feeling before, when I was a kid. It wasn't a girlfriend, it was my mum. I was one of eight children. My mother always told me she didn't have time for me, that I had to look after myself because there were so many younger children for her to look after."

He started to sob, but carried on talking through his tears. "She's tried to apologize to me many times because she feels so guilty about the way she treated me … but I've never been able to forgive her. She would never pay any attention to me. I was always afraid she was going to abandon me completely."

Ian sobbed uncontrollably as he recalled the pain. I put my hand on his chest over his heart. "Yes," I said, "that makes sense, there's the feeling. Let yourself feel it now. Give it some room."

Ian had touched on the wound which pushed people away. Desperate for closeness, he also distrusted and feared it because of the pain and fear of abandonment he held in his heart. As the oldest child with an absent father, circumstances had forced him to take the place of his dad in the family but without the attention he so desperately needed from his mother. He felt both abandoned and betrayed by his mother, and later in life the pattern repeated itself in his intimate relationships. Part of the problem was that when he did open himself, all the rage and hurt from previous disappointments came flooding back — and in particular, the anger he felt towards his mother for her rejection of him.

Of course, he was not fully aware of this anger, which had long since been repressed but people could sense it when they were around him. Since unconscious hostility is difficult if not impossible to hide for too long, no doubt his women friends were well aware of it too, and would have felt unsafe around him. So they closed down or backed away to protect themselves, in effect repeating his mother's betrayal; and in turn, their withdrawal fuelled Ian's rage and despair, adding to his wound, and justifying his belief that women could never be trusted.

## BETRAYAL AND THE BROKEN HEART

It is apparent to me now that some of us can never have what we deeply want until we explore the broken-heartedness and sense of betrayal lying at the centre of our being. There is a point in intimacy when the heart begins to open and we begin to trust. And it is just then that the ancient rage that defends us rouses itself, and the anguish of previous betrayals is likely to pour out.

The experience is so common, we might do better to expect it. Yet the last thing most of us expect is to become the object of the rage of someone else's wounded child and we usually simply shut down to protect ourselves. Thus the scenario repeats and repeats: we get into a relationship and just when it is beginning to become intimate, it falls apart.

Awareness of our sexual wound might not change the feelings we have, but it might well change what we do with them. People carry this wound for a long time — without ever becoming aware of it — continually disappointed and betrayed by a succession of untrustworthy partners, never finding a solution, never realizing the extent of their own wound. They may talk to numerous counsellors but never be able to make a significant breakthrough to change their pattern of behaviour.

## BEYOND MIND, INTO THE BODY

One reason this wound remains so hidden — in spite of access to all kinds of practitioners — is because we rarely get into the body sufficiently to move the energies involved. We may talk *about* a problem but rarely will we attempt to explore it directly. Talking about problems is fine as far as it goes but as long as "mind and body", or "love and sex" are split, talking is usually insufficient. It tends to be a cerebral affair, and while much understanding may ensue, the split continues as before. With the talking approach, healing can take a long time, or be deferred indefinitely. *At some point we have to get into the body to heal the body.*

As Ian discovered, the process of entering the void experientially can be a powerful tool to help unlock the secrets of the sexual wound. Of course, he was earnest, and well primed by previous therapy. As long as we are willing to engage the process with some sincerity, significant results can come quite quickly.

Ian was aware enough to immediately grasp the significance of what he had encountered in his bodywork. He had released the full force of his rage and related it to a childhood wound rather than to his girlfriend, who no doubt was dealing with her own wound in her own way.

"Why don't you write to Leslie and let her know about what you've learned through this process," I suggested to him one day. "When she hears that you are exploring your rage and owning it rather than blaming her, she may be willing to re-establish a relationship with you."

"It makes sense," he had to agree.

"And even if she doesn't respond," I went on, "at least you'll know you've done everything you could, and maybe you'll be better able to let it go and move on."

Whether she responded or not was not the issue. The important thing was that Ian address the situation and get on with his life. During the bodywork and breathing, there had been so much energy coursing through his body that Ian finally became aware how much of his chronic fatigue was due to the repression of feelings he could neither understand nor acknowledge. He had also realized that he had actually been coping with a lack of vitality for years before his accidents had pushed him over the edge and forced him to acknowledge it.

"It's like a huge weight off my shoulders," Ian said. "I've had this knot in my stomach for years on and off, and I've never known where it came from or what to do about it."

Ian's appetite returned and his stomach settled down; and he was much less anxious and far more energetic. And he did write that letter to Leslie. She responded and they met and talked. She admitted that she had always been afraid of his anger and felt threatened by it when their relationship had started to become really intimate. Their conversations did not bring them back together, as too much water had passed under the bridge but through the process Ian was able to come to a much deeper understanding of his own part in what had happened between them.

Ian's wounding is not at all unusual; I'm sure many people can recall similar agonies. For some however, the initial wound is compounded by physical or sexual abuse or other significant trauma with the result that later in life they experience much more intractable symptoms. A history of such sexual trauma is unfortunately quite common in people who have chronic pain.

# Chapter 10

## SEXUAL ABUSE

*The great problems of life*
*– sexuality, of course, among others –*
*are always related to the primordial*
*images of the collective unconscious*

— Carl Jung

*T*he issue of sexual abuse is becoming increasingly public, a frequent subject in the newspapers, on radio and television. Childhood abuse and its legacy to our societies is emerging in our collective awareness after centuries of suppression and denial, though it is probably much more widespread than many people realize.

Studies have shown that while an alarming number of women report childhood abuse, men are also learning to reconsider — and daring to bring to consciousness and report — their experiences. It seems that often men's conditioning has encouraged and rewarded them for viewing heterosexual childhood abuse as "seduction." Moreover, any traumatic sexual encounters they have had with men may be doubly difficult to speak out about in our still deeply homophobic society. It is for these reasons that some researchers are beginning to consider that men abused as children may eventually register more psychological disturbance than women.

It is of course mere pedantry to attempt to measure or compare the kinds and degrees of suffering inflicted on children by adults who for whatever reason feel compelled to involve them in sexual activity. Such "scientific" pronouncements must surely be no more than another way to avoid the real discussion. It is a tough issue; none tougher perhaps. But to really grapple with it, we must return to the dynamics of our collective sexual wound and our society's manifestations of what I've called the love/sex split.

If the people who sexually abuse children were drooling cretins or wild-eyed outcasts with whom we had nothing in common, we could perhaps deny any personal responsibility for the problem. But the truth is not so comforting. Abusers, we now know, are "ordinary" people from all walks of life with the single distinguishing feature that often they have themselves been abused.

Sexual abuse, it turns out, is not the preserve of a handful of extraordinarily disturbed adults but looks rather more like the tip of an iceberg of cruelly suppressed and distorted sexuality in our society as a whole. When we look deeply into the issue, we may begin to understand that the sexual abuse of children is really the manifestation of the enormous collective wound, the sexual wound we all carry. Indeed, "they" might be said to be no more than a dark side of "us" — an expression of our collective shadow, a part of us we would rather not acknowledge.

The wound is now so old, we are often completely unconscious of it and pass it from one generation to the next, through father-daughter/ mother-son dynamics. It tends to produce opposing energetic distortions in men and women — leading to endless misunderstandings between the sexes. While by no means a universal rule, men tend to respond to abuse by closing off the flow of energy to their "heart," as if denying to themselves its existence; while women tend to close down the pelvic area — again, as if they wished to deny it and its too-frightening memories. And both sexes tend to believe it is the other sex that "has a problem."

## FATHER-DAUGHTER SEXUAL DYNAMICS

Freud's so-called "Oedipus" and "Electra" complexes describe family triangles in which the child takes on the burden of the sexual energy of the parent of the opposite sex. When men are disconnected from their inner female (or "anima"), they may unconsciously manifest the negative or shadow side of the father archetype. They may be emotionally distant, overly rational, and intellectually rigid; and they may subject their children and partners to "discipline," justifying their violence with the argument that it's "good for them." Unfortunately, many men suffer this fragmentation, finding it difficult to express their emotions and often able to connect with their feelings only through sexual contact. When their "heart" is closed, sex may be the only available vehicle these men have for the expression of their emotions.

Women — particularly those with the opposite imbalance of a weakly developed inner masculine principle ("animus") — may be initially attracted to such men because they can appear strong and decisive and project an air of confidence. However, they will soon become disenchanted if they cannot connect with them on a heart level. If no emotional rapport develops, the couple's sexual relationship generally deteriorates, and the man's only route to expression of feeling becomes blocked.

At this point, the relationship might well end. In those relationships which continue, affairs, addictions or violence could enter the picture; and where there are children, the stage is set for father-daughter abuse.

Rather than connecting to his feminine nature, the father projects an idealized female onto his daughter. The daughter, who may have suffered from such a father's emotional distance, will generally respond happily to his attentions, willing to oblige him in return for the affection and attention she has lacked. Often she will not understand the abusive nature of their relationship and in any case, sadly, she can't usually do much about it.

If the relationship becomes overtly sexual, the daughter may feel her love and trust betrayed literally unspeakably — for she will likely not be able to speak it — particularly if any violence is involved. Later on, as a woman, she may find she closes down sexually with men she respects, while being strangely attracted to men who are abusive. Her need to defend herself against betrayal by men she respects may lead her to initiate relationships with men who don't deserve her respect.

## MOTHER-SON SEXUAL DYNAMICS

Something similar can occur between a mother and her son, although the abuse is less likely to be physical and more likely to be what has been termed "psychic incest." Those women who are disconnected from their own masculine energy may unconsciously behave in a way that is psychically invasive — for example "nagging," or always wanting to know what the son is doing, feeling, thinking — while at the same time expressing a distaste for normal sexual expression. Rather than connecting to her inner masculine nature, such women often transfer their desire for a heart connection from their husbands to their sons; and the sons of such mothers grow up with a not-so-subtle sense of their mother's censure of their sexuality, while experiencing a continuous "phallic" invasion (at the heart level) by their mother's unconscious animus.

In such situations, the growing son must deal with the contradiction between what his mother says and what she does. When he is older he may find that he has internalized such negative attitudes and experiences guilt and shame around sex, unless it is impersonal. Or he may assume, defensively, that any woman who will have sex with him must be a slut.

The irony is that need to defend against psychic incest is one of the things which leads a growing boy to close his heart. He learns very young that it is dangerous to trust women, since the one woman he most trusted has betrayed him. Later on as a man, if he cannot open his heart to a woman, he may attract her psychic invasion — a desperate attempt to force the intimacy he cannot allow — as he pushes her away.

## CLINICAL SYNDROMES

Few people who have experienced sexual abuse in childhood come to a physician with the information directly. Usually, the memories have been repressed and lie behind layers of physical armouring, so that the only clue to their presence is the body's muscular tension. Those people who do remember may feel embarrassed or fearful of voicing their memories, or may fail to see any relevance to their adult lives. Add to that the collusion of most physicians — who are often so uncomfortable discussing sexual matters with patients because of their own wounding that they would rather avoid the subject altogether — and the fervent wish of society in general not to have to examine such upsetting information, and it is not surprising that many victims remain silent and even unaware. The sexual abuse of children, in particular, is such a difficult issue that physicians, who do not usually have any relevant training they can call on, may feel helpless and unwilling to become involved. They may also have difficulty in believing their patients' stories.

However, the body can sometimes recall things the mind would rather forget, and bodywork techniques have altered our understanding of the sources of illness for all time. Suddenly, people are "reading," in graphic detail, traumatic childhood sexual experiences from the imprints those experiences have left on the body-mind, and have no idea what to do with the knowledge so acquired. How does one integrate unacceptable memories when the only strategy one has developed is to forget? As more men and women come to bodywork for inner healing, the ramifications of exploring repressed memories will continue to unfold.

## ENERGETIC DISSOCIATION

When a part of the body is damaged, the mind may try to "numb out" the injured part by withdrawing its attention from the area. The familiar experience of favouring an injured leg to avoid pain is a crude physical example of dissociation. As we favour the injured leg, we put more energy into the good leg, which bears the greater part of the physical load. This strategy works well as long as the body heals quickly, since the dissociation is temporary. Energetic dissociation becomes a problem however when pain is chronic, or when the mind uses it to avoid facing an original trauma.

*A vicious circle is established when a dissociated area won't heal because in time the fact of dissociation rather than the injury becomes the primary hindrance to the healing process.* Any part of the body can become dissociated, but in our sexually wounded society, the pelvis has become a prime area of dissociation for many men and women.

The specific illnesses which arise can be understood from a reading of the energetics. Where there is significant sexual wounding, the mind withdraws from the pelvic area. Energy is diverted from the pelvic organs, and relocates in the upper part of the body, the chest, the upper back, and the face. The result is excess energy — heat, or tension — in the upper body and a corresponding coldness in the lower body, abdomen and pelvis.

Symptoms which might result from such an imbalance are legion. Excess upper body energy could result in neck and shoulder tension, headaches, anxiety, insomnia, susceptibility to colds and sinusitis, acne, hyperthyroidism, breast lumps, hypertension and/or heart disease, unremitting menopausal flushing, and some PMS symptoms. Concurrently, the lack of energy in the lower body might be behind symptoms as diverse as irritable bowel syndrome, urinary incontinence, low back pain, dysmenorrhoea, menorrhagia, and PMS symptoms, recurrent urinary tract infections, interstitial cystitis, and infertility; in men — stroke, heart attack and impotence might result. In either case, the hot above/cold below clue can alert the physician to the possibility of sexual wounding or abuse, even if they are not mentioned by the patient.

Of course, a reverse energetic distortion is perfectly possible, though it is less likely to be associated with abuse. The endemic nature of the love/sex split means that virtually everyone is likely to be affected in some way by sexual shaming. For example, excess energy in the pelvis might be a contributing factor in lower back pain, prostatic enlargement, ovarian cysts and fibroids, while a deficiency of energy above could lead to angina.

Even more fascinating, perhaps, is how our cultural imbalance might be tied to modern illnesses such as chronic viral fatigue syndrome and AIDS. Sexual activity can critically deplete a person's energy, eventually leaving them seriously fatigued and putting their health at risk. Over time, such depletion may compromise the immune system, making them increasingly susceptible to a variety of viral illnesses which might otherwise be harmless.

If the sexual activity is also promiscuous, the risk of sexually transmitted diseases — or STDs, including AIDS — may also increase. That is not to say that everyone who gets an STD is sexually wounded but the energetics are certainly worth considering. Nor should the analysis be interpreted moralistically. Sexual activity itself is not the "cause" of disease but it may well be a relevant factor in any condition in which there is low energy or weakened immunity.

What to do about it is another matter. Many of the above mentioned disorders are exceedingly common and are treated in a matter-of-fact way by physicians. It would be as outrageous to suggest that everybody with one of the above complaints was sexually abused as a child as it would be foolish to ignore the possibility of abuse in a person who had inexplicable recurrent symptoms in those areas with a significant hot above/cold below energetic imbalance. If we understand sexual abuse to include sexual shaming, it is quite likely that these common problems are in some way related to society's collective wound.

Healing in this area is not a matter for a ten-minute office interview. Only extensive and in-depth explorations of repressed and denied feelings can free up the blocked energy so it can be recovered and integrated, and create an awareness in us which will prevent us from transmitting the wound to the next generation.

## GISELLE : UNHEALED KNEE LIGAMENT AND ASTHMA

Giselle was a 45-year-old asthmatic who came to us after injuring her leg at work. It had appeared to be a relatively minor injury, a strained knee ligament which was expected to be back to normal in a few months. But for some reason Giselle's ligament never healed. In fact, it got worse and worse, despite physical therapy. Naturally, her physician was concerned and referred her to an orthopaedic surgeon who suggested an MRI scan. Everything was normal; and since he couldn't see a cause for her pain, he suggested that Giselle undergo arthroscopy, a procedure which allows a surgeon to look inside the knee.

Giselle ended up having two arthroscopic examinations of the knee at different times but there was never anything of significance found to explain why she was in so much pain. Next she had a bone scan, which showed nothing; and this was followed by serial cortisone injections and regional anaesthetic blocks. But nothing seemed to help her at all.

When Giselle arrived at one of our retreats, she was walking with a cane, was unable to bear weight on her sore leg or move it much at all. Her knee bent little more than ten degrees from the straight position. She had managed to stay at work and be productive, something which was very important to her but by the end of the day she was exhausted, going home only to sleep. She managed to overcome the pain in her leg by unconscious dissociation, using her mind to simply block out whatever it could not handle, in a way that is similar to the heart and pelvic blocks of the sexual abuse victims we have just been discussing.

When Giselle became extremely fatigued, she found that her foot would start to shake uncontrollably. She also found that it was sometimes difficult for her to get to sleep at night because the leg would begin shaking just as she was dropping off.

ENERGETIC FRAGMENTATION

Despite being able to cope, Giselle was in sufficient discomfort that she was more than willing to explore her pain to see what she could learn. What she discovered, however, was shocking and took her far beyond her physical pain into experiences she had long since pushed out of her consciousness.

When Giselle took her first fearful step into the void, her right leg began to shake in just the same way as it did when she was trying to sleep. After a minute or two, the other leg began to shake in a similar fashion, and soon hands and arms joined in. This was nothing out of the ordinary. The peculiar thing was that the movement of the various limbs seemed disjointed, as if there was no connection between her arms and legs and body. Shaking, Giselle seemed fragmented and compartmentalized, as if her limbs were separate entities.

Later, however, both legs began not only to shake and tremble but also to squirm, as if she were trying to get away from something. She was immensely strong and would kick away any one who attempted to get close to her. The leg movements were so violent that unless she consciously decided to shut them down, they continued even after she left the acupuncture room.

Later still, Giselle described a feeling of being smothered, as though something was pressing on her chest, and she had such difficulty breathing it seemed as if she were being choked. Further exploration of this choking brought to the surface a memory of being sexually molested. Though who the molester was was not immediately clear, as we addressed the pressure on her chest, it gradually softened and Giselle began to cry, tears of regret and shame which had been bottled up in her since she was a child.

Giselle had always had difficulty sustaining a relationship. Single and forty-four years old, she thought she had chosen her aloneness, but when questioned she had to admit it was not what she deeply wanted. Her difficulty in relationships seemed to stem from a terror of her own sexual feelings, which were accompanied by a sense of suffocation and of imminent annihilation. The moment she opened her heart to anyone, those feelings would surface and threaten to overwhelm her. Attacks had been sufficiently violent to land her in the emergency ward, where she had been diagnosed with asthma; and over the years she had slowly but surely become a prisoner of these feelings, convinced that it was best to live her life alone.

In fact, what was really going on was not so much asthma, although it may have masqueraded as such, but a deep distrust of her own body, the compelling need to avoid all intimate relationships, and an inability to allow her sexual energy to flow freely. She had closed her pelvis and walled off her heart to prevent further damage but she lived with a torment she could not describe to anyone. The tension in her body was enormous.

## INTERPRETATION OF INNER EXPERIENCE

When sexual abuse memories surface in bodywork, the desire for revenge can block further healing. One way to get around this is to remember that images which surface during bodywork represent an *inner* reality and reflect inner states and repressed feelings, not necessarily actual "events" in the everyday world. Like dreams, these memories can be intense and omnipresent but it is crucial not to draw hard and fast conclusions. If we interpret memories produced through bodywork too literally, we will get caught up in trying to explain them rather than just releasing the blocked energy and moving on.

Giselle had to face exactly this issue. When memories began to surface during bodywork, she might have been tempted to seek revenge on her abuser rather than focus on healing but fortunately she was able to maintain the focus on herself. We have seen others take the path of revenge with disastrous results to their health. The letting go required for healing means just that: letting go of everything.

## BREAKING THE WALL OF FEAR

During one later session, Giselle had a breakthrough. She entered the void and shortly arrived at the place of suffocation. The feeling intensified as she became visibly short of breath and an asthmatic wheeze developed. There was a sense of someone's hand around her neck and a feeling of panic accompanied by the desire to get away; but this time Giselle stayed with the process. I mimicked the sensation she had described by pressing on her chest as she went deeper into the terrifying experience.

Very soon after, while she was still wheezing but able to talk, I took the opportunity to speak with Giselle about the positive attributes of her pain, how much it had taught her about her sexual wounding, and how it had opened the doors to intimacy again.

"One characteristic of a good friend is that she sticks around when the going gets rough," I suggested to her. "Can you see how nifty it is that your pain has stayed around long enough for you to learn these incredible things?"

"Yeah, right," she agreed sarcastically. "You're joking of course."

"Not really," I replied.

"You're nuts! crazy!" Giselle exclaimed. But then she started to laugh. She laughed, and then she laughed some more, and before she knew it, she'd stopped wheezing and was breathing as freely as if there never had been any problem. "Nifty!" she howled. "That's funny!" And she laughed some more. She was through to the other side and the constriction in her chest was gone.

Giselle never forgot the word, and she soon discovered that just the thought of it was enough to break her breathing restriction and allow her to stay in situations from which she would otherwise have run. She felt like a new person, and was more determined than ever to continue the healing process and make her life more to her liking. As of this writing, the pain in Giselle's leg remains but her attitude toward it has shifted fundamentally. She now considers her pain a teacher and is willing to learn everything that teacher has to offer her.

MERYL : RECURRENT INFECTIONS

Giselle's journey was protracted and her story continues but with adequate preparation, appropriate intention and a supportive context, healing from sexual abuse does not have to take forever. Meryl was a forty-year-old woman who had chronic recurrent vaginal infections, abnormal cervical cytology, pain with intercourse, and ulcerations in the vagina following inter-course. She had run the gauntlet of regular treatments: she had been dosed with multiple courses of antibiotics; and she had undergone several investigational procedures, including colposcopy, cervical biopsy, and laparoscopy. Several years of her life had revolved around treatment of her ongoing pelvic com-plaints.

After attending a number of personal growth courses, Meryl realized she might have been a childhood victim of sexual trauma and finally decided to explore her illness through acu-puncture and bodywork. When I saw her, she was well prepared and ready to face any demons that might surface during the work; and she was keen to get started. In one session, Meryl re-experienced being raped as a young girl by a trusted family member. Within a few weeks, the physical problems that had plagued her for twenty years cleared up, and she was able to enjoy a renewed physical relationship with her husband.

The sexual wound is so common that in some measure or other it is an issue for everyone. Abuse simply intensifies the wound and adds to the shame which is already present. And though society still seems to want to sweep the issue under the rug, I believe denial is no longer desirable, or even possible. Awareness of our wounding can bring about a new and more honest relationship with ourselves and our bodies, recover much lost energy and give us renewed vigour for living.

# Chapter 11

# THE GRAIL

*The central issue of the healing journey*
*Which stops all but the most committed*
*Is that the task involves healing*
*A wound which won't heal*

Several years ago, someone sent me some Qi Gong[1]
tapes. They seemed interesting, but for some reason got put
aside. A couple of years later when I was having a particularly
bad time with my back and was despairing of ever finding relief,
I happen to hear about Qi Gong from some colleagues and took
them out again.

I watched the tapes and early one morning decided to
walk up a nearby hill and try out some of the postures. Having
reached the top, I took off my shoes and socks and started
through the various positions I had learned, slowly and me-
thodically.

After a few minutes, I became aware of a very faint desire to
move my hips and pelvis. I felt supremely self-conscious and
exposed on the top of the hill at sunrise and checked to make
sure no one was watching me. The only people around were
early birds doing the rounds with their dogs. So, eventually,
when I felt sufficiently alone, I let my hips move.

Within moments, the movements had become rhythmical
and almost effortless pelvic tilts. I checked once more to make
absolutely sure no one was watching then let the movement
develop as it wanted, feeling my lower back and pelvis loosen and

1. Qi Gong is a discipline involving different postures and exercises designed to build
and move energy in the body.

a warm surge of energy flow up my back. It hurt a lot, but felt good too, and I could feel something letting go.

I completed the set of exercises and walked down the hill, astonished to find that for the first time in five years I had absolutely no back pain. While I knew that these spontaneous movements were a part of Qi Gong, their real meaning was lost on me until I experienced them personally. The inner urge and the reluctance to let go, I later realized, signalled the doorway to the void.

I was naturally very happy to be free of pain but I felt humbled and slightly chastened, too. It was immediately obvious that I had to rethink the meaning of my symptoms in the light of the kind of movements which seemed to relieve them. It was clear I had a frozen pelvis, and I finally recognized that my back pain involved something beyond the mechanical explanation I had offered myself.

## THE WOUNDED HEALER

In the normal scheme of things, the patient is considered to be sick and the physician well. The doctor relates to the patient for the sole purpose of diagnosing and treating the patient's illness. Ideally, the treatment cures the illness. The physician's own spiritual health — and the "background radiation" of our society's psychic wounds — are considered irrelevant to the healing process.

Such are the assumptions of modern medicine. But our profound psychic wounding cannot be so easily dismissed. Its nature is such that it transcends the boundaries between patient and physician and destroys any imagined distinction between the two. To deal with another's wounding adequately, a practitioner must be fully aware of her personal wound and how it manifests. The physician's spiritual integrity is vitally relevant to any healing relationship.

How can we understand such a hidden wound if no one can see it? One way perhaps is to turn to mythology. A similar wound has been a central theme in several myths, and one story which illustrates it well is the story of the Holy Grail.

## THE GRAIL LEGEND

One of the best known of the many variations on the Grail story was left unfinished by its author, Chretien de Troyes, in the late twelfth century. His version of the story begins when an arrow pierces the groin of a young prince, the future "Fisher King," and cannot be pulled out again. The tip remains in the wound, and the wound suppurates and will not heal. By the time the prince is king, he is unable to stand, and spends his days languishing on a litter in his castle in constant and agonizing pain while the land for miles around his castle withers to an utter wasteland where nothing will grow, and famine and disaster sweep his kingdom.

Strangely, the castle of this same benighted King contains a living miracle. The Holy Grail, the cup from Christ's last supper, is carried every night in a procession in the castle's banquet hall. Three maidens dressed in white walk through the hall, the first carrying the platter which held bread at the Last Supper; the second, the lance, which pierced the side of Jesus on the cross; and the third the Grail, still full of the blood which fell from that wound.

The Grail of legend shines with a mysterious and blinding light and has the power to heal anyone who drinks from it — anyone, that is, except the Fisher King. He, it turns out, can only be healed by an innocent young man, who must ask two vital questions. The first is, "What ails thee?" and the second, "Whom does the Grail serve?"

The task of healing the Fisher King falls on the young Arthurian knight, Sir Percival (or Parsifal in German). Percival was born in Wales in some obscurity to a widowed mother who had deliberately moved to the country to bring up her son away from the attraction of the life of knights and jousts. Her husband and two older sons all lost their lives as knights and she was determined to protect her youngest from the same fate.

But Percival, whose name means innocent fool, is still little more than a boy when a chance encounter with some knights galvanizes his attention and he decides to leave his mother to become a knight himself. She is heartbroken and pleads with him, but it's no use. Eventually she blesses him, wishes him well, and makes him a homespun garment to remember her by. She cautions him to wear it at all times, to treat women with respect, to go to church daily, and not to ask too many questions.

And so, Percival leaves home and soon meets a mysterious, huge and rather fearsome knight in red armour who directs him to King Arthur's court at Camelot. When he arrives at court and asks to become a knight, however, Percival appears so ridiculous in his country outfit that one of the ladies of the court bursts out laughing.

It turns out that this lady has not laughed in six years and legend had it that whoever made her laugh would be the finest knight of all. So, King Arthur makes Percival his knight and sends him on the quest for the Grail. He tells him that he can have the horse and armour of the Red Knight if he can find him again and take them from him.

Before long, Percival encounters the Red Knight again and, by some inexplicable circumstance, manages to kill him. He puts the giant's red armour on over his mother's homespun garment, and rides off excitedly on the knight's enormous steed — only to realize that he is totally out of control. The experience suggests to him that there is more to knighthood than the gear, and he realizes he needs a mentor.

He finds his way to the castle of the knight Gournamond, who instructs him in the arts of knighthood and tells him what questions to ask when he eventually finds the Grail. He also suggests that it is time Percival takes off his mother's homespun garment.

Percival eagerly takes on the quest for the Grail. He earns a reputation as a fierce fighter, winning many jousts and battles along the way. Then, one day, he gets lost in a forest and chances upon a lone fisher in a boat on a lake. Percival asks the man where he might stay the night as it is getting rather late. The fisherman tells him he is welcome to stay at his castle, since there isn't anywhere else nearby. He tells him to go down the road a little way, turn left and cross over a drawbridge. Unbeknownst to Percival, this lone fisherman is none other than the wounded Fisher King whose castle contains the miracle he is seeking.

Grateful for his hospitality, the young knight dines with the king that evening and observes the strange procession. Although he is familiar with the Grail legend, however, he forgets Gournamond's instructions and instead avoids asking any questions as his mother had counselled, contenting himself with small talk and idle chit-chat instead.

In the morning, he wakes up to an empty castle, saddles his horse and sets off. Once he crosses the Fisher King's drawbridge, however, the Grail castle disappears and he finds himself once again lost in the forest. Meanwhile news of Percival's heroic deeds has found its way back to King Arthur, who invites him to return to Camelot for a celebration of his great deeds. But the rejoicing is brought to an abrupt end by a hideous old woman who rides into the court on a decrepit mule, reciting all Percival's misdeeds.

She recounts all the misery and suffering Percival has caused through his conquests and accuses him of having failed to ask the right questions of the Fisher King. Percival is horrified as he remembers the quest that was entrusted to him and recognizes the opportunity he has missed. Chastened, he heads out on his quest again but cannot find his way back to the Grail castle, and wanders about, year after year, jousting and rescuing maidens, struggling to remain chaste and remember his task.

But over twenty years of fruitless searching, he becomes more and more bitter and disillusioned and once again forgets his quest until one Good Friday he meets some pilgrims who ask him why he is armed to the teeth on such a holy day. Suddenly, Percival remembers and, filled with remorse, accompanies the pilgrims to a hermit for confession. The old hermit hears his story and directs him to the Grail castle once again.

The story by Chretien de Troyes seems to break off here, prompting many others to try their hand at an ending. But perhaps it is really up to each of us to finish the Grail legend for ourselves. For instance, let's look at the story from the point of view of the healing journey, and try to identify the main characters as part of an individual consciousness.

## THE GRAIL AND HEALING

If we understand the Fisher King to be the spiritual body, the story tells us that this spiritual body carries a wound which won't heal. Second, the wound which won't heal is in the groin, indicating that it involves sexuality, generativity or creativity. That the wound might be both spiritual and sexual in nature is the key to the meaning of the Grail myth.

The young knight, Percival, on the other hand, might represent youth and innocence, the part in us which acts before thinking, leaps before looking, which feels it is invincible. The homespun garment, that relic from childhood, might represent our attachment to our mothers and the difficulty we have in learning to care for ourselves — in both senses of the term —

instead of expecting others to do it. The Red Knight is clearly a hero figure, the image of manhood to which every youth aspires; the hideous hag, as she points to Percival's failures, may make her appearance as people grapple with chronic pain. And the Grail itself, being shaped like a uterus and carrying blood, might be the inner feminine, which has the power to heal.

The compelling message conveyed by the Grail legend is that healing is available to anyone who asks the appropriate questions but that for some reason we forget to ask these questions as we get caught up in life. The story also speaks clearly to the wounded feminine. It speaks to the repression of the emotions, the sexual wound, and the difficulty of opening the heart. Being archetypal, it refers to the collective feminine, not the personal, which is to say that its message applies to women as well as to men.

## THE VISIBLE WOUND

The most obvious wound we have is the one which brings us to the physician in the first place. That wound might be causing us pain or manifesting any one of an infinite variety of other symptoms. Acute and self-limiting conditions do not usually prompt us to ask deep questions but chronic complaints eventually make it clear that, like the Fisher King, we have a wound which won't heal.

Quite frequently, our wounding is perfectly obvious to family, friends, and even casual acquaintances but is not obvious to us, who sit languishing and groaning in agony like the Fisher King, waiting to be made well. It can take many years before we realize we have such a wound as we go from pillar to post looking for the elusive cure. Some people never realize it, and live out their lives in quiet desperation. Chronic pain then, wherever it is located, can serve as a pointer to the deeper "Fisher King wound."

PAIN SPEAKS

My own chronic pain began in my lower back, very much the area of sexuality. For many years, I had been acutely aware of unresolved sexual tension but preferred to see my back pain as largely a mechanical problem — the result of too much squash played with a damaged leg — rather than seeing the deeper issue involved.

No doubt the mechanical problem existed. It always does. Squash was always my big love, the great joy of my life; and a lot of my self-esteem was tied up in competing. Winning on the squash court was like beating the Red Knight in a joust. I would spend hours taking out my frustrations in hitting a little black ball as hard as I could against a wall, and trying to prove I was something by beating other people. I felt if I could win on the court, I was a worthwhile and important person.

Of course, time marches on, and eventually the demands of a sport begin to tell on the body. For those who can let go gracefully, it may not be a problem, but craving the image of the Red Knight can be a difficult thing to relinquish. I only considered quitting when, at thirty-five, my back was so painful I could hardly tie my shoelaces, let alone play squash competitively. It was a difficult time; without squash I had no outlet, nowhere to put my excess energy, and I felt frustrated and frightened about what was happening to my body.

As my back pain plagued me increasingly, I was forced to stop pushing myself physically but it never occurred to me to enquire about the deeper wound I might be carrying. It was not until I began to study the energetics of sexual wounding that I realized I might myself be a classic example and understood that my over-exertion on the squash court had simply been the catalyst of a pre-existing imbalance. My denial had lasted quite a long time.

The truth is, my sexual wound is as great as any of my patients', and I owe my understanding of it largely to the work I have done with people who have chronic pain. I feel deeply grateful to them: their bravery and commitment to healing has allowed me to see my own pain more clearly. Like many people, I longed, deep down, for a satisfying intimate relationship but was not really willing to open my heart sufficiently to connect emotionally with my partner. I experienced my feelings through sexuality, and had the classic energetic imbalance of excess below, deficiency above: that is, energy diverted from the upper chest stagnated in the pelvis, manifesting as high tension, which predisposed me to injury there. Of course, because I could to some extent relieve the tension through intercourse, I had little reason to explore the problem more deeply until the sexual connection in my marriage deteriorated, and I had to wonder why.

## THE EMOTIONAL WASTELAND

In addition to my general angst, I found myself as I reached my late thirties, increasingly incapable of feeling anything at all, and I retreated further into my intellect as a way of avoiding an inexplicable emotional desolation. Happiness seemed to have fled my life and I felt increasingly grey, barren and joyless. I had become the Fisher King; and though the Grail appeared at my table every night, in the form of a loving family, friends, work and all the material comforts, nothing touched me.

I could feel no reason to celebrate anything. Birthdays, Christmas, parties, family occasions, nothing could make me feel anything other than a deep, flat greyness which I watched gradually engulf everything in my life. Initially, of course, I blamed outside influences, such as my job as a physician, my wife, my family, difficult patients, finances — you name it — since I could not see that I had any kind of problem.

But in the end I had no-one to look to but myself. Like the kingdom of the Fisher King, my life had gradually became a wasteland, and although I seemed able to help other people with their problems, there seemed to be nothing available to help me. One way to forget the greyness was to work harder, so workaholism became a way for me to escape the pain. At least there I thought I was doing something useful, paying the bills, and getting the recognition and approval I so desperately needed to bolster my self-esteem. So I filled my days with appointments and projects and began to spend less and less time at home. When I was home, I became increasingly difficult to live with — frequently monosyllabic, and often shut up in my room meditating, or reading — anything to be emotionally unavailable, while my anger grew inside me like a tumour that invaded every part of my psyche.

## BODYWORK

It was into this depressing milieu that my discovery of the healing power of bodywork and acupuncture came. My first encounters with Traditional Chinese Medicine were serendipitous. When I began, on a hunch — I might have called it mere curiosity at the time — to use acupuncture on whiplash patients, I had no idea I was intuitively turning towards a path that would teach me to heal my own wounds and open my heart.

Slowly, I began to understand that medicine did not have to be practised the way I was trained to practise it. It occurred to me that here was a light in my darkness — at least at work. A whole new world of alternative medicine opened up before me, and I found real passion, excitement, and an outlet for stagnant energy. Acupuncture demanded and rewarded intuition and openness; and it had a playful, creative quality which conventional medicine as I had practised it had ground out of me. The more I learned, the more I felt inspired and sustained by what I was encountering.

Perhaps it was my age, and my growing fear of the "wasteland" of my heart. I don't know. But I do know that from those first encounters, the experiences I had and the people I met allowed me to gradually probe the deep-seated wound which lay in the darkness of my own soul. And like Percival, back at the Grail castle for the second time, I began asking some real and pertinent questions.

## WHAT AILS THEE?

First, I had to ask, What ails thee? Ironically, "What ails thee?" was exactly the question I had been asking patients for an eternity without realizing that a more meaningful act might have been to turn the question on myself. And it was the deep message of some of those patients' experiences that eventually drove home the answer to me. They clearly spoke to a primary sexual wound and it began to dawn on me that my back pain, my joylessness and my difficulty with my relationships were really all just different aspects of the same thing.

The second question, "Whom does the Grail serve?" seems to speak to the healing power of the inner feminine. At least one writer has interpreted the Grail as an archetypal image of the eternal feminine, since its shape, contents and implication of new life suggest a uterus. Without a connection to the feminine, an individual remains heartless. The Grail represents what is lost when we live too much in our heads, severing our connection to our inner female or anima.

It began to seem to me that healing must come from the heart; that it was like a kind of aware compassion; that there was no place for the "hands-off" distance I had been taught; that in fact the fear and denial that distance concealed blocked any possibility of deep healing. But it was only when I began to actually open my heart a little at work, and found myself crying with people as they entered the dark night of their pain, that I realized that here, in the engagement of profound healing, was no place for my precious "objectivity" or my "detachment," any more than it was for the person seeking to regain their whole-ness and health.

Several years into these exciting discoveries, it dawned on me that it was time to bury the hatchet and begin to fully com-mit to my marriage, something I came to realize I hadn't really done before. I had mouthed the words alright but my mind was usually elsewhere, fantasizing about the wonderful life I could be having somewhere else with somebody else. And although physically present, I had been the quintessential absent father. I'd been at home in body but not in spirit nor mind nor heart, and I hadn't been any fun to be around during my children's growing years.

Today, I still struggle with my wound. But at least I can say I am learning to ask myself better questions. And I live with an awareness of my wound and tend to deny it less and less.

## TWO ENCOUNTERS

The Grail myth suggests that we often stumble into the Grail castle early in life. During the teen years, or even younger, there is often a chance exposure to the archetypal feminine as we dream of what we could do with our lives. If we do not ask the right questions then — and there is very little chance that we will — we leave the experience none the wiser, and spend years in the wilderness looking for meaning in life through heroic deeds and achievements. After all, learning a trade, or climbing the ladder of success are really just the modern equivalents of fighting duels and searching out dragons!

It is only much later in life that we get another chance at the Grail. Some disenchantment with the way we are living, or perhaps an illness or chronic pain, will enter our lives and signal the arrival of the hideous hag. If we will listen to her, she wastes no breath in pointing out that we have forgotten our real quest, and sends us back out on the search. And by this time, tired of fighting duels or saving the world, a humbler and wiser person may come to the Grail castle and begin to ask some more meaningful questions. The second time, we may be more inclined to ask, "What does it mean? Why am I sick?" In this way, difficult experiences can become opportunities for us to rediscover some meaning in our lives.

Interestingly, even if we make it back to the castle and pose some meaningful questions, the story seems to suggests that there may be no concrete answers. Perhaps it even suggests an answer is unnecessary or even undesirable. The question is the answer, the search is the discovery, and the Grail is found when we live the question as the central motivating force of our lives. In my own life, the decision to live the question was the most terrifying yet at the same time most exciting project I have ever undertaken.

From the perspective of the collective consciousness, medicine's scrupulously rational approach, which seeks to explain everything without reference to fundamental human emotions, and its denial of a sexual wound in patients and physicians alike, leaves the therapeutic milieu looking very much like dinner at the Fisher King's castle. Although the Grail is right there in front of us, and has the power to heal, it seems few of us ever dare acknowledge it, or ask meaningful questions, contenting ourselves with superficial chit-chat — perhaps because the deeper questions would involve the taboo subjects of emotions, sexuality and the spirit. I hope before too long we mature sufficiently as a society to return to the castle with a change of heart.

Part IV

───────

JOURNEYS

*into*

HEALING

# Chapter 12

# THE SLEEPERS

*He who learns must suffer. And even*
*in our sleep pain that cannot forget*
*falls drop by drop upon the heart,*
*and in our own despair, against our will,*
*comes wisdom to us by the awful grace of God*

— Aeschylus

*I*t always surprises me how different the healing journey is for each person and how our experiences in the void clearly reflect those differences. Naturally, the energies which arise from the void — anger, sadness, grief, joy — are common to everyone but the journey itself is unique to each individual as we recapture a sense of the selves we lost when we built our persona to function in the world.

Void experiences are also often astonishing in their simplicity and directness; and when we learn to observe them without interference, judgement or attempts at problem-solving and rationalization, we find ourselves at the heart of the heart of things and can tune in to the mystery of our existence.

## INSOMNIA REVISITED

A long-standing psychic wound may disturb any physiological function to produce symptoms of chronic illness. The clients whose stories I want to relate in this chapter suffered distortions of their sleep rhythms. Both had relied on medications to counter their symptoms; and in both cases, the knowledge required for healing arose spontaneously in a thoroughly convincing way.

In our society, many people are chronically sleep deprived. We live in a world of high stress and our lives often demand far more from us than is healthful. Some of our excessive activity is forced on us by circumstance but probably a lot more than we realize comes from our wounding, which makes us so unsure of own worth that we overachieve compulsively, hoping somehow to justify our existence.

My medical training was a case in point. Hospital interns and residents were expected to work several days in a row without adequate rest. So while we were supposed to be delivering health care to the public, our own health was being routinely compromised. Such an obvious contradiction of values was rarely raised as an issue — partly because no one dared buck the system, and partly because sleep deprivation was seen as a perverse sort of rite of passage.

Of course, physicians are not the only ones who are stressed out and short on sleep. In our society, sleep deprivation is nearly universal. And it doesn't go away. Over time, as people sacrifice themselves to achieve their goals, fatigue may precipitate as illness. Most of us, then, would feel a lot better if we could just let go and rest for a while. But while deep rest is almost always beneficial, too much rest can also be a problem. Some people use sleep to escape, or feel constantly fatigued though they have plenty of potential energy. In such cases, sleep may be being used as an avoidance or denial of a wound.

## TIM : CHRONIC PAIN AND INSOMNIA

Tim was a thirty-six-year-old man who injured his hand in an industrial accident. He had had multiple surgeries to repair his thumb, including two tendon transfers, and a fusion of the metacarpo-phalangeal joint. But in spite of the success of these operations, he was left with stubborn chronic pain and had come to rely on large doses of medications to control it.

Before his accident, Tim had been extremely active. He seemed to have a real liking for dangerous occupations such as logging and oil-rigging. Many years previously, he had had half his face smashed up in a logging accident, an injury which required extensive surgical repair. But other than some difficulty sleeping, he claimed to have recovered from the experience, so it was curious that the apparently lesser thumb injury should have stopped him in his tracks. There had been no improvement over three years, and Tim was becoming more and more depressed and unproductive.

Tim was a wiry fellow with sharp features and the hint of a smile, which only showed on the rare occasions he wasn't focusing on his painful thumb, which had become an all-consuming concern. He wore a wrist splint at all times, and during my initial examination refused to allow me even to touch the thumb. But the thing which really struck me about Tim at our first meeting was his red eyelids, and the way he kept rubbing them as if trying to keep himself awake.

Tim was keen to explore the different bodywork techniques we offered but because he was loath to have his thumb touched, I explored the areas near his facial injury during our initial acupuncture session instead. It all seemed simple enough but no one was quite prepared for Tim's encounter with the void. When the first needles went in, he made a lot of noise; and then, with very little warning, passed out cold. I tried talking to him but there was no response. He had vanished somewhere into the hidden recesses of the void and seemed quite determined to stay there.

After an hour or so, Tim came to and looked around as if he were in a totally foreign place.

"What's going on?" he asked. "Where have I been?"

"I'm not sure," I answered truthfully. "You seemed to be very sound asleep. I suggest you take it easy getting up as you will probably be a bit wobbly."

Returning from the void to normal consciousness takes some time and people often think they are fine, only to find they are quite shaky and cannot walk properly. It can be quite a frightening experience.

"I'm okay. I'm quite okay," Tim insisted as he got up — far too fast for my liking. "I think I'll go have a smoke and a cup of coffee."

"That's fine, Tim. But if you don't mind I'll go with you just in case — you may be more unsteady than you think." Tim was extremely wobbly, though he had no idea how unstable he was. He put on his shoes, walked out of the room, and started up the stairs. But he hadn't climbed more than three steps when he put his hand to his head and began to sway back and forth.

"Whoa!" he said. "I *do* feel a little strange."

Then he seemed to turn to jelly. He collapsed into my arms and was gone again. Nothing we did could rouse him.

I felt a little surge of panic, the physician within me saying, Help! What's going on? What should I do? But at the same time another part of me felt certain that this was all part of his process and that he would wake up when he needed to. So we carried Tim to a couch and let him sleep.

Tim slept for more than a week without ever really waking up other than to eat or have a smoke. He slept and slept, day after day, in an unusually deep way. We chose not to interfere even though it seemed most odd, and after ten days — as if on cue — he woke up.

The change in Tim was remarkable. He looked completely different, as if he'd finally got some beauty rest. His eyes no longer looked red, and the infectious smile began to show up more and more.

"You know," he told us, "I've been in so much pain, I haven't really slept in ten years — ever since my face was crushed by that log. It feels so good to sleep again!"

Tim went home for a couple of months and then returned. He was fascinated by what had happened and was now curious to understand more. He was clearly much more alive. His depression had lifted and his eyes were much less red, and he was keen to do more work.

With some deep breathing, facial pressure and manipulation of his thumb — which he now permitted — Tim started the familiar myoclonic shaking which signalled his entry into the void. His injured hand began to shake violently, and then he passed out just as before.

Over the next few days, we helped him enter the space over and over again, until he was able to get there and begin to maintain some awareness of what was going on. Gradually, he came to understand that he was revisiting the accident in which he had been knocked unconscious, and was re-experiencing his coma. Could it be, we wondered, that over the years his body had fought unconsciousness so vigorously that even sleep had seemed a threat?

Tim learned fast. His experiences spoke loud and clear to him and he began to grapple with a deeper wound — the one which drove him into such dangerous occupations in the first place, the one which perhaps lay behind everything. The eldest of four children, Tim had taken on the role of father at the tender age of seven after his parents separated. As a result, he never really had a childhood.

His mother gave all her attention to the younger children and let Tim take care of himself. Nothing he did seemed to merit her attention. Tim learned that to be accepted was to be completely self-sufficient; and, as an adult, he therefore pushed himself to exhaustion, always picking the roughest, toughest jobs — as though still craving her recognition and lacking the mechanism to give it to himself. The image he projected was the machoist of the macho. He had to be the best.

As Tim slowly woke up, he came to understand how deeply fatigued he had become over the years; and as a result of his void experiences, was able to begin to reverse the process. The amazing thing was that as he got more rest, he noticed his left thumb pain diminish, and it was not too long before he was able to throw away his splint.

When I ran into Tim two years later, it was clear he was a changed man. There was a sparkle in his eyes. He was running his own very profitable business and was lively and enthusiastic about life.

## DIANA : CHRONIC FATIGUE

Animal bites can be dangerous. While the punctures are often tiny, they can occasionally become seriously infected. Physicians consequently tend to be cautious and prescribe antibiotics early.

Diana was a 36-year-old woman who had developed chronic and disabling fatigue some two years prior to coming to see us. She had been working as a veterinarian's assistant, a job she loved, when one day she was bitten on both wrists while restraining a cat. The bites did not seem very severe, no more than scratches she thought, so she went on working despite a strange numbness up one arm. Later that same day, however, she became quite dizzy and then passed out. Her employer called an ambulance and she was taken to the nearest hospital where the wounds were dressed and she was sent home. But the next morning her arm began to swell and she went on to develop a nasty infection which required hospitalization and six weeks of intravenous antibiotics.

Though the infection eventually responded to treatment, Diana had never really recovered her previous energy. She developed intermittent fevers and swollen glands. She seemed to have entered a downward spiral to total exhaustion. She found herself sleeping up to eighteen hours a day without feeling refreshed and eventually became unable to function. Two years went by and nothing changed.

Naturally, Diana sought medical attention and was diagnosed with a variety of conditions from sympathetic dystrophy, to chronic fatigue syndrome, to depression. The fact was there seemed to be nothing physically wrong with her: her blood tests were normal; there was no sign of any serious illness; no anaemia or diabetes which might cause fatigue.

But in the end it made no difference. Diane seemed to have checked out. She was fatigued for no identifiable reason. Her physicians eventually threw up their hands and the inevitable referral to psychiatry left her wondering if she was crazy.

When I first saw Diana, I found she could carry on a conversation alright but seemed strangely "spaced out" and lackadaisical. She still took pride in her appearance but didn't seem to have interest or enthusiasm for much else. It was as if she was not quite fully present. She said she felt different from the other people and couldn't relate. In particular, she had difficulty being with people who were in pain, and almost wished she had pain of her own just so she could feel something, and perhaps be understood.

I wondered what could possibly have so knocked her off her centre. She obviously had no idea; and while we hoped a thorough exploration of the void would sort things out, I also wondered if she wasn't actually living in some kind of void. Maybe she needed to get out of the void, not more into it. I really had no idea.

To make matters worse, her acupuncture sessions produced no movement, no myoclonic shaking, nothing. Diana was thoroughly disgruntled.

"Why aren't I shaking like other people?" she asked in despair. "What's wrong with me?"

I didn't know, of course, but didn't want to discourage her, so I tried to give her a broader understanding of what we were up to.

"Everybody's healing journey is unique," I explained. "Do you really want someone else's journey, because if you could have it, you would have to have their problems too. For example do you really want Laura's pain? or Kenneth's, or Joe's?"

"No, I suppose I don't," she answered reluctantly. But I knew she wasn't convinced. In a way, she *did* want someone else's journey. At least other people could "feel" something. And she desperately wanted to feel something — anything.

In spite of her lack of myoclonus, or other visible sign of entering the void, Diana seemed to warm to the community, and by the time she left us she was feeling much more energetic. But within days of returning home, she was back to her old excessive sleeping. Mind you, there was not much for Diana to go home to. She lived alone with her dog, and had no family to speak of, and no vision of anything different.

"I don't think I'll ever have a relationship," she had said on several occasions. "Men can't be trusted. Much better to have a dog. They are always there when you need them."

It was strange how Diana had never really engaged in life. She lived by herself, had no relationships except with animals, had stopped working, and now was hardly ever awake. And even when she was awake, she wasn't really there, but seemed to exist in some far-away dreamy realm that no one else could get to.

I enquired a little into her past.

"I never knew my birth parents," she told me. "I was brought up in an orphanage and adopted at the age of five. I found one of my half-sisters a couple of years ago but when I enquired after my mother, I was told she'd died. There were other half-brothers and sisters but I've only met the one. We all had different fathers, so I have no idea who my birth father was, or is."

Then, with a bit more animation, she added, "There's a chance I might find my dad though. I'm trying to trace him by the surname my mother left on my birth certificate. Something might come of it, I suppose."

She told the whole story matter-of-factly, without much emotion, as if it were someone else's story. No doubt she had been separated from her family so young she didn't remember.

Since there had been no response to acupuncture, I decided to inject the cat-bite puncture sites with a little xylocaine. The idea of injecting xylocaine into trigger points is quite commonplace in Europe, where it has become known as "neural" therapy. In a way it is similar to acupuncture, with a little added punch of pushing energy into the sites which have been damaged.

It was a long shot, but I felt there was little to lose. One of the ideas behind neural therapy is that puncture sites can develop into energetic foci which remain indefinitely, and continue to upset the body's equilibrium in unpredictable ways. "Resetting" the disturbed foci with local anaesthetic might just allow the body to begin healing. Nothing ventured, nothing gained, I reasoned.

I was not to be disappointed. No sooner had I injected the smallest amount of xylocaine into her right wrist than Diana swooned.

"Oh wow, oh wow!" she exclaimed over and over.

She tried to stand up but almost immediately fell back into her chair. "Oh wow," she repeated, incredulously. "This is like drugs — without drugs!" Her shoulders began to twitch with the first signs of myoclonus I had seen in her.

"This is awesome!"

Indeed, I thought. Still, I had no idea what it meant or where it was leading. The next day Diana asked to do it again.

"What is going on?" I asked. "Is anything interesting happening?"

"It's really weird," she replied slowly. "I seem to be recalling events in my life from when I was a baby. Right now, I'm about three years old. I can see it, taste it, smell it, everything. It's like I … like I missed it the first time 'round."

"What do you mean 'missed it'?" I asked, genuinely mystified. "I mean, you've lived your life, or you wouldn't be here to talk about it."

"Yes, of course," she agreed. "But I don't think I was in my body. I mean, I don't exactly know where I was, but I wasn't there. I was, like, gone somewhere else. I've never really been here. Now it's like I am living my life for the first time."

I was amazed. For the next few days, we watched Diana slowly go through her whole life from age one to twenty-four. For much of the time she seemed in another world, even though we could talk to her quite freely.

When she had reached about twenty-two, Diana again alluded to other people's experience.

"I wish I could feel what Laura feels," she said.

I felt myself going for the answer I had given her several times before when I stopped in my tracks. There were tears in Diana's eyes, tears I had not seen before. It was the first sign of emotion I'd seen in her.

"What are you feeling?" I asked gently. "Why don't you let that feeling come? That feeling which is there right now."

"I don't know," she groaned. "It's just that I don't feel anything — or I don't know what I feel — I can't put words to it."

I could see she was very close to her wound, and I had a sudden inkling of what it might be. Of course she couldn't put words to it. The wound was probably pre-verbal. She had been taken out of her mother's arms and sent to an orphanage long before she could talk. One can only imagine what an infant must feel who has such an experience. It would have no words for alarm, abandonment, distress. Perhaps to cope with her abandonment, Diana had abandoned *herself* somehow, had left her body, had refused to "be" with her adoptive mother. Certainly, she might choose to avoid all human relationships, in order not to be abandoned again. I put it to her.

"Perhaps," I said as gently as possible, "you were too young to put words to the feeling of abandonment you must have had when you were taken from your birth mother."

The remark hit home. Emotion seemed to flood into Diana as though from some unseen well. She started to sob, her shoulders heaved and her whole body shook as it responded.

"I feel hot all over," she told me as she wept uncontrollably, repeating, "That's it — of course," over and over. "Now it all makes sense."

Diana had abandoned herself to cope with the pain of her abandonment as an infant. As an adult, she had been driven by a feeling she could never contact directly which told her never to risk deep commitment again. Instead, she had taken comfort in animals. She lived and worked with them; and when it was time for her to recover herself, it was an animal which initiated the events which led to her self-discovery.

Diana left us feeling energetic and keen to get on with her life. But her enthusiasm changed to fear as she came face to face with the reality of her situation. There she was, thirty-six years old and just waking up to herself. She had no training, no degree, very little income, and no particular interests, no idea what she wanted to do with herself. Like Rip van Winkle, she had been "away" for a long time and the world had moved on.

A couple of months later, she returned to see us. The spontaneous review of her life which had been moving along smoothly since she left, had suddenly stalled as if in mid-sentence.

"I was doing so well, then all of a sudden it stopped," she lamented.

"How old were you when the process stopped?" I asked.

"Twenty-six," she said. "I know I need to complete this process but it's stopped and I can't seem to get it started again. What's more, no one seems to understand what I'm going through."

"Has your energy been holding up?" I asked hopefully.

"You know, it really has," she exclaimed. "I've been jogging forty-five minutes every morning."

"Okay, things could be worse then. It can be difficult to keep up the healing process away from a supportive environment," I reassured her. "Safety is a big issue for you, you know. Did something scare you?"

"Something sure did," she affirmed. "There was a fire in the building where I live. Right afterward, everything just stopped — like a big wall came down. Its been really frustrating — I wonder if a bit more xylocaine would do the trick."

I injected a bit of xylocaine into the scar from the cat bite. "Oh, wow!" she gasped, just like the first time. "That's got it going!" Her shoulders stared twitching and her left leg began to shake.

"I can feel energy moving up and down my stomach," she said. Then she added, "You know, I think I've been absolutely terrified. Most people have sorted things out by the time they are thirty-six. I'm only just beginning my life, and I'm not sure I can do it." Of course she would be frightened, I thought.

"It's pretty rough for you right now isn't it?" I agreed. "You have to decide if you want to live in your body, and it doesn't feel at all safe. There is probably no safe place for you to be since the only place you know is out of your body."

"You're right," she said. "I have nowhere I can call home. My dog is all I have."

Diana faced a life-and-death decision. Coming back to life meant being responsible for herself, finding something to do with her life, meeting and interacting with people, feeling, and learning to trust — and she wasn't at all sure she was up to it. Yet despite these misgivings, I felt certain she had already made her decision.

"There has already been a shift in your spirit," I reassured her. "I think the inner change has already occurred. And if that's in place, the outer changes are bound to happen, probably sooner than you think. If you can just trust and keep your eyes open, something will happen before too long."

Diana eventually returned to her veterinary job but was put out on the front desk away from the animals she loved. She didn't like it but felt she had little choice until something else showed up. At first, she thought she would like to assist other adoptees who were looking for their birth parents but her initial enthusiasm was dampened by the amount of training she would need to enter the field professionally; and, deep down, she knew she wanted to work with animals.

Diana's life review had convinced her beyond doubt that her life had meaning and purpose. However, discovering what that purpose was was going to be a challenge. Nothing but working with animals had ever really excited or motivated her and she needed to find something which would excite her sufficiently or the pressure to simply abandon herself again would be too great. In a way, her story is just beginning. As of this writing she is still looking.

# Chapter 13

# ARCHETYPES

*It matters not what our ultimate fate is*
*So long as we face it with ultimate abandon*

— The Teachings of Don Juan

*W*hen we enter our void, we often express personality traits or behave in ways which seem quite unrelated to our ordinary, habitual ones. Most commonly "shadow," or unexpressed, aspects of our personality will come into view, though occasionally people adopt dramatically different personas.

Over time, too, it has become clear that these shadow traits are often eloquently expressed by our symptoms; and that these symptoms are therefore *necessary* — are what is missing or denied in our being and therefore a vital part of our wholeness, without which we can never be well.

The following story illustrates such a situation.

## MARLA : BREAST CANCER

Marla came to me via Mary Joan after undergoing a mastectomy to apprehend the cancer in her right breast. An axillary node dissection had also found two locations in her armpit where the cancer was beginning to spread. Further, Marla's tumour was "oestrogen receptor negative," meaning that it carried a slightly worse prognosis and was less likely to respond to chemotherapy. Marla's oncologists had nevertheless recommended that she undergo adjuvant chemotherapy and radiation anyway, as it is the standard procedure. But before they could begin, she decided to explore her alternatives.

Marla went to counselling, joined a cancer support group, took megavitamin therapy, selenium and beta-carotene, tried naturopathic herbs, took Essiac (a herbal preparation which has been claimed as a cure for cancer), went on a macrobiotic diet, and eventually came to see us. She was obviously taken by surprise when Mary Joan pointed out that she might be overdoing things a bit. In Marla's view, it was only smart to try everything.

I always feel vaguely uneasy when I see people pursuing alternatives as aggressively as Marla because I've come to understand that it is often this intensity which has made them ill in the first place. If this imbalance is not changed, then nothing else will fundamentally change, including their health. It's tragic to see people put huge efforts into healing when the effort itself may be a symptom of the problem.

When I explained to Marla that whatever I might recommend might make things worse, she told me that while she was aware of her "driven" tendencies, no one had ever pointed out that they might be part of the landscape of her illness; and she was curious to explore what that might mean.

## THE SHAMAN AND THE SAMURAI

During her stay with us, Marla began to sing, chant and dance spontaneously in sessions like an elderly shaman. Over ten days, her dancing and chanting became so intense she felt she had "become" the old man. And her conviction was transpersonal: others around her had the impression that they were in the presence of an old medicine man.

In other sessions, Marla made sounds and movements suggesting a Japanese samurai. And similarly, during those experiences, she felt she had "become" the samurai and, again, people around her experienced the force of his presence.

While these startling experiences might seem to have little to do with breast cancer, their effect on Marla was profound and far-reaching. She understood them immediately and deeply, for they were archetypes which expressed her various "primary patterns," or life themes.

## ARCHETYPES AND LIFE THEMES

Archetypes match the stages of our lives. The primary female patterns are the daughter, the young woman, the mother and the crone; and the primary male patterns are the son, the young man, the father and the old man. These archetypes can be expressed positively or negatively, in a balanced or an unbalanced way, depending on whether our individual spirit is fully expressed, or distorted. The archetypes have symbolic rather than literal significance. Because they are not intended to replicate social clichés but to form a matrix of human capacities and potentials which are available to both sexes, we will refer to them as "it" rather than he or she in the descriptions that follow.

## THE SON

The son archetype represents an idealistic and exuberant energy. It is the adventurous, curious, inexhaustible phallic energy which tempers the self-importance of the authoritarian and rigid father energy. When balanced, son energy brings a lightness and newness to life situations which our father energy would tend to make heavy and oppressive. When imbalanced, son energy manifests as a Peter Pan, or Puer Eternus attitude — an irresponsible fun-seeker, careless of the destructive potential of its disregard for others.

## THE YOUNG MAN, OR WARRIOR

The young man or warrior archetype represents daring, conviction and risk-taking. It focuses the natural exuberance of the son energy on a goal. When balanced, warrior energy retains individuality, heart and creativity. It represents hope for the future and constructive change. When imbalanced, it becomes automaton-like, both heartless and mindless, cynical and without individual expression, like the soldier who takes orders blindly and becomes capable of carrying out atrocities without feeling or a sense of responsibility for his actions.

## THE FATHER

The father archetype is that of a protector and leader. It represents the teaching we seek in order to cope in the world and take care of ourselves; and the authority, order, convention, and rational thought which represent the "world stage" on which our external lives are played out. When imbalanced, this archetype manifests as heartlessness, cruelty, oppression, rigidity and conformity. The energy of the father archetype needs to be allied to the heart, or it can produce a tyrant.

## THE OLD MAN, OR SAGE

The old man archetype represents wisdom acquired in living, and the maturation of other masculine energies. It manifests as a balance of restraint and exuberance, discipline and joie de vivre. It represents the maturation of the curiosity implicit in the son energy in a deep understanding of life which accepts contradiction and can keep conflicting forces in balance. And it manifests the maturation of the father energy as reasoning used in the service of human connection. Equally, it is the maturation of the warrior energy as the capacity for ethical and intellectual focus which can also be flexible when the situation requires it.

When balanced, old man energy is clear and understanding, the epitome of wisdom. When imbalanced, without heart development, it may use its skills and understanding in the service of its own ego; or allow the intellect to deteriorate into cantankerousness and childishness.

## THE DAUGHTER

The daughter archetype manifests as eager relation, compassion, devotion and connectedness. It is the energy of the unknown which seeks to be known and to know; the energy of sexuality which can both fascinate and frighten. Daughter energy when balanced is the energy of uncalculating and happy rapport between self and others. When imbalanced, it manifests as manipulative and attention-seeking, exploitive and destructive.

## THE YOUNG WOMAN, OR WOMAN WARRIOR

The archetype of the young woman, or female warrior, manifests as the energy of the activist. When balanced, it is powerful and connected, manifesting as heart energy fully in touch with phallic energy. When imbalanced, it may be entirely predatory, using sexuality impersonally. The imbalanced warrior energy sacrifices intimacy and closeness, and may forego relationships altogether, or have many.

## THE MOTHER

The mother archetype represents trust in life, unconditional love, nurture and protection. When balanced, maternal energy supports individuality and nurtures potential. When imbalanced, it withholds nurture, retards potential, or attaches conditions to love, thus compromising its offspring's potential to thrive in the world. Just as the unbalanced paternal energy is the result of a lack of connection to heart energy, unbalanced maternal energy is the result of a lack of connection to phallic energy. This negative maternal energy is the archetype of individuals who are unable to connect to the world, and who fulfil their emptiness by living vicariously through others.

## THE OLD WOMAN, OR CRONE

The old woman archetype represents loving wisdom and profound intuition. It epitomizes mature heart energy and inner knowledge which has remained connected to phallic energy, realizing a balance of intuition and generativity. Sometimes called "the crone," the old woman archetype lies hidden in a society which gives its whole attention to youth and beauty and whose fears lead it to disparage old age and champion selfishness and thoughtlessness. When balanced, the old woman energy is intuitive and wise. When imbalanced it can be exceedingly dangerous since it is powerfully connected and knowing, and can destroy those who are unwary.

## MARLA'S ARCHETYPES

The rational mind might have some difficulty with the notion that a medicine man or a samurai could be relevant to breast cancer. Nothing could be farther removed from the world of surgery, chemotherapy and radiation. But such is subjective reality, and such are the ways in which the body communicates, unique to each individual. In fact, Marla's projected archetypes need only make sense to her for there to be a meaningful connection and the possibility that an experiential understanding of her own repressed energies would fundamentally affect her health.

Perhaps the shaman represented the energy of the wise old man, and the samurai, that of the young man, or warrior. Until they surfaced in their archetypal forms, Marla was not fully conscious of these energies inside her, so if she expressed them at all it would be largely unconsciously. Perhaps her aggressive approach to life reflected unconscious warrior energy, while the energy of the wise old man came through in her social work, where her role might have been similar to that of a tribal elder. Since she became more conscious of these energies through exploring her cancer, one could say that the problem and the solution were the same.

Marla's remission continued for a few more months, and as time went on she began to think she really had beaten her cancer. The disease had become a secondary issue after she uncovered her shaman and warrior energies, and as her remission continued with no sign of recurrence, she decided to return to her busy and responsible job as a social worker. Within a few months was totally caught up in her old life — a life mainly devoted to looking after others, to the detriment of herself. Unfortunately, a few months after returning to work she found a second lump in her armpit and came back to us in a panic.

Now, more than ever before, Marla needed to draw on those energies she had discovered. It was a difficult time. She was aware that her chances for survival were now radically slimmer, statistically, and that she was now in real danger of losing her life to her disease. It was tempting to take the view that she should have had chemotherapy, but that had never been an issue. Marla really wanted to face her illness consciously and wanted our guidance.

I did not know what to say or do but fortunately Marla volunteered her own answer.

"I know why my cancer has returned," she said with conviction. "I got so absorbed in this process that I slipped right back into denial. ... I pretended to myself I was cured and stopped looking at the reality of the situation. ... That's why I went back to work. ... It wasn't a smart thing to do ... I know. ... Because it's not really what I want to do with my life."

"Well, what do you really want to do then?" I asked, intrigued to hear what she might say next.

She looked up at the ceiling, as if musing over her options. "I think I'd like to go to Germany."

"Why Germany?" I countered, wondering what she was really thinking. She paused for a moment, and then when she continued, I'm sure it was the shaman who spoke.

"Well, I don't know how much time I have left," she said slowly. "What I would really want to do is finish what I started ... to explore alternative cancer therapies, and perhaps write about them ... there's a couple of clinics in Germany I've always wanted to check out but I've not been because of my various commitments ... and the cost was high enough that I told myself I couldn't afford it. But now ... what the hell have I got to lose?"

"Marla," I cut into her thoughts for a moment. "Have you really heard what you just said ... I mean ... really heard it?"

She stopped suddenly as if struck by an insight, looked directly in my eyes, and announced, "I know what to do now."

The next we heard from Marla was a postcard from Germany. She had gone to a European nutritional cancer clinic and really felt she was on the right track for the first time in her life.

Six months later, Marla was gone, but she had lived vibrantly until twenty-four hours before her death when she had a sudden stroke from cerebral metastases. She had found time to write about her experiences, and had prepared a small manual of alternative options which cancer patients could pursue. To my mind, she had met her destiny in a vital and creative way.

I was fortunate enough to attend her funeral where several hundred people turned up to pay tribute. In a moving eulogy, Mary Joan pointed out and confirmed what many people intuitively felt, that Marla had left this world as healed as anyone could be. Dying is something we all do and surely any medicine which merely tries to prolong life is missing the point. True medicine means discovering who we are, why we are here and what we are meant to do. It has to do with living more fully, not longer. Those were attributes which Marla had amply demonstrated.

# Chapter 14

# POWER ANIMALS

*The desire to take medicine*
*Is perhaps the greatest feature*
*Which distinguishes man from animals*

— Sir William Osler

Stories of power animals accompanying people as guardian spirits have always fascinated me. In West Coast native and shamanic traditions, people call on and welcome animal energies into themselves. When illness comes and personal power is lost, a shaman might understand the loss as the loss of a power animal. The shaman's task is to journey in the psychic realm on behalf of the person who is ill to retrieve the lost energies.

Shamanic traditions consider that animals represent specific characteristics. A wolf has the energy of a wolf, a lion the energy of a lion, and so on. Though I had long been fascinated to read about such subjects, I had little direct experience of them until I attended a weekend workshop focused on techniques for exploring our inner worlds.

At one point in the workshop, we undertook a guided visualization which began with a walk down an imaginary garden path. The imaginary path went along through a meadow and eventually arrived at a gate which opened into a garden. At this point, our guide asked us to visualize an animal's face on the gate.

The task seemed simple enough so I looked at the gate and vaguely imagined the head of a wolf. I'd always been attracted to images of wolves but my visualizing skills were tested to their limit as I tried to piece together its teeth, tongue and ears.

Next, we were asked to open our imagined gate and go into the garden. That also seemed simple enough. But when I tried to get through my gate, I found it impossible to get past my wolf. Our eyes locked and I felt unable to follow the rest as they were led elsewhere by the visualization guide.

"Oh heck," I thought, "I can never visualize very well."

Suddenly, I noticed that my wolf had changed. It was no longer a mask on a gate but a whole living animal standing right next to me. Though part of me had been anxious about "catching up" with the visualization, another part of me knew I was right where I should be.

There was a wolf standing near me and I felt a tingle of excitement. My wolf was very male, large and shaggy and seemed quite savage. I felt a little frightened but also understood at some level that this wolf was a part of me. I also knew, from working with other people, that I must embrace this projection.

So I did, literally. I walked up to the wolf and hugged him, embracing him as if he were a member of my family. Then, without any warning, the most extraordinary thing happened. The wolf and I began to come together. I had the sensation of the wolf coming into my body, merging with me.

At one point, he got stuck. I screamed in frustration as his forelegs struggled to get into my arms, and his haunches into my lower back. But at last we were united. I felt a surge of power and "wolfness" — the sense of running wild and free on the plain — and wanted to howl. My whole body tingled for hours.

I've learned to respect such experiences, which occur in the void quite frequently, and to watch for them in clients.

## TREVOR: HIP INJURY AND WOLF ENERGY

Trevor was a fifty-five-year-old man who lived in Northern Alberta. He had been a farmer all his life, working the wheat fields from dawn till dusk, until one day he fell off his tractor. Unable to

move, he was taken by ambulance to hospital where he under-
went surgery for a fractured right hip. He recovered but never
regained his former physical capabilities or self-confidence and
suffered from intractable low back pain.

Never one to turn down a new experience or opportunity,
Trevor willingly entered the void to find out what would happen.
After a few minutes, he seemed to go off somewhere in his mind,
as if he were not fully present. Shortly, he began to snort, lick his
lips, and rub his head against me like a puppy wanting attention.

His behaviour seemed almost contrived, so for a few minutes
I had to consciously reserve judgement. Then Trevor began to
howl. The next thing I knew, he was down on all fours, roaming
the room like a young dog, occasionally nudging Mary Joan or me
and trying to lick us all over. It was quite amusing, though neither
of us particularly enjoyed the licking.

Trevor returned from the void with no conscious memory of
what he'd experienced and was quite astounded to hear us talk
about the puppy he had become. But the reason he was astounded
was not what we assumed. In fact, quite the opposite.

"You know, my wife has told me I behave strangely at night
sometimes," he told us quite matter-of-factly. "I thought she was
making it all up but what you've told me more or less matches."

I asked Trevor what she meant by his behaving strangely,
and he answered quite candidly.

"She knows about this puppy you're describing — actually
it's a wolf cub, she thinks. She's told me about it. I thought I was
just sleepwalking or something. I do have a recurring dream
about a wolf cub but I had no idea I was acting it out." Then
Trevor had an idea. "Do you think we could tape the next session
so I could take it home to Evelyn?" he asked. "I think it might
answer a lot of questions she has."

So the next day we took a tape recorder into the room and put
it on the window sill just above the mat where Trevor would be

lying. I wondered whether anything would happen with this kind of surveillance in effect but we weren't disappointed. Trevor's wolf cub showed up on cue and filled the small room with howls and barks, playing and sniffing around us for a good half hour. The tape must have been hilarious.

A couple of months later, Evelyn and Trevor both participated in a program. At one point, I talked to Evelyn about her husband's experience.

"He makes all kinds of funny noises at night, kicks and snorts and moves around in the bed," she said. "It was impossible to get any sleep at night with all his goings on, so we've been sleeping in different rooms for years. I always wondered what it was all about. I used to think perhaps he was crazy, you know."

"What did you do about it?" I enquired.

"Nothing. It was just very odd, and I didn't feel comfortable talking to anyone about it. I couldn't bring it up with the family doctor. Besides, Trevor thought I was making it all up and just denied everything. I would have been the one they thought crazy, you know. So I just put up with it. After I got over the initial shock, it seemed pretty harmless."

Trevor and Evelyn had lived with this unusual phenomenon for years without ever being able to talk about it to anyone, or even to bring it up seriously with each other. When they had discussed it, she had wondered whether he was crazy, and he had wondered whether she had made everything up. Over the years, they had let the matter drop but it was one of those things that both would have liked to understand. The simple experience in the void, and the validation which the experience brought to both of them, had much more impact on Trevor's pain than anyone could have predicted.

Both Trevor and Evelyn had many good laughs over the whole issue, and perhaps as a result they visibly lightened up during the period they were with us. Indeed, Trevor relaxed so much that by the time he left us, his chronic back and hip pain had all but disappeared.

PAUL : BACK PAIN AND BEAR ENERGY

Paul was a thirty-year-old First Nations man who had injured himself falling off a ladder one day. He felt something go in his back and was unable to finish his shift. He limped around for several months waiting for his back to right itself before being diagnosed with an L5-S1 disc injury and a spondylolisthesis (a slipping forward of one vertebrae over another because of a weakness in the bone) requiring surgery.

Unfortunately, the operation was unsuccessful — the fusion did not take on the left side — and Paul continued to be in a lot of pain. Although he had been offered further surgery, he was reluctant to risk it when the first operation had not helped.

Because Paul's job involved a lot of heavy lifting, he could not return to work and wanted to move on to something else. But there were few opportunities for a man with little education and chronic back pain. By the time he came to us, he was taking a disturbing amount of codeine-laced pain killers and had become morose about his future. He'd found little support in his home community and his life seemed to have come to a full stop.

Though Paul was keen to do anything he could to improve his situation, he was frightened at first and reticent about what we suggested he do to help himself. It turned out he had had an extremely difficult childhood. He was the third child and first son in a family of ten. His father had been alcoholic and Paul had suffered a lot of physical abuse as a result.

During the first session he was so apprehensive I could hardly touch him. Whatever I tried, he would say it was too much. He asked me to stop very early in the session, saying he'd had enough. I honestly wondered if he would stay long enough to get anything out of what we offered. But by the second day, something had changed. Either Paul had decided to trust us or to trust himself. Either way, he very quickly settled down and jumped right into the void with amazing gusto. This time, he kept telling me to work harder and dig deeper.

Some time into his third day with us, Paul sought me out to tell me he had a monster headache and wondered if I could do anything about it.

"It's right at the top of my head," he said, pointing to the centre point at the vertex, right in the middle of the top of his head.

"That's strange," I thought. The vertex is an unusual place for a headache.

"Trigger points" are often associated with chronic pain syndromes. They are generally located in tense muscles in and around the painful area and may be useful as acupuncture points in treatment. Most headaches are triggered by tender points found in the sub-occipital area at the back of the head, or in the temple area. I had, in fact, found two such tender spots behind his head at the back in the more common location just the day before and had put a couple of acupuncture needles back there to try to release the pain, without success. I thought we might as well try the top of the head as anywhere else.

Now the point on the top of the head has tremendous significance in Traditional Chinese Medicine. In TCM it is known as "Hundred Meetings," and is referred to as an "ancestral point." One way of understanding the point is that it refers to the hundred ancestors, the power of the wisdom and knowledge of parents, grandparents and beyond. They are called to meet and help the patient in his distress.

I am never quite sure what these things mean till an experience confirms or illustrates them but they have an uncanny way of revealing themselves. As I inserted the needles, I told Paul about the meaning of the point with the intention of facilitating a connection to his roots. We had worked with many First Nations people and found that they had often lost a meaningful connection to their spirit. I had every reason to suspect that Paul might have the same problem. I put the needle in and sat back.

Almost immediately, Paul began to shake and shiver as if the room had all of a sudden gone cold.

"What's happening?" he demanded as he started losing control. "Oh ... Oooaah ... Aaaah ... Ooaaaaah ... Wheee!" he cried. "I can't sit here. I have to get down on the ground."

With that he got down on all fours and arched his back as the energy coursed through his body, shaking him to the core. Then he started to make a different sound. An unmistakeable growl, at first slow and low-pitched, grew louder and more insistent until after about five minutes it filled the room. Paul raged at the top of his lungs and began to scrape at the ground, bending his finger tips like claws and gouging the carpet.

"I feel like a bear!" he cried. "My hands feel like claws! I can feel the power! I don't believe it. I don't believe it!" he yelled in obvious excitement and awe.

I felt tremendously excited as well and wanted to join in the ruckus. "Aaaarggh!" I cried in unison, hoping to encourage Paul to let go even more.

"Aaarggh!" Paul shouted as he pawed the floor leaving even deeper gouges in the carpet. It was an impressive display and the energy of an animal was clearly in the room with us. But more was about to happen.

Paul looked up over into the corner of the room for a moment. "I see a light over there. It seems like it's calling me — what is that? ... What is that?" he exclaimed, repeating the question several times.

I hesitated, wondering what was going to happen next. Paul crawled quickly over to the corner of the room where there was a large oak desk and a heavy bookcase full of books. Between the

bookcase and the desk was a small opening leading into a cub-
byhole in the very corner itself. Paul turned around and backed
into the corner, all the while growling and roaring and pawing
like a bear. Then, he lifted his arms sideways into the furniture.
The oak desk shifted two or three feet as if it weighed almost
nothing and the bookshelf went crashing to the ground. Later,
two of us found it difficult to move them back.

Paul stayed in the corner several minutes, raging away at
the top of his lungs and pawing the ground before gradually
settling down. Then he collapsed into a heap on the floor.

As he gradually returned to normal consciousness he exclaimed, "Wow, I've never felt so relaxed. What happened?"
When I explained to him what we had seen, it was immediately
obvious to Paul he had come into contact with a power animal.
Though he knew of such things in his culture, he had never had
such an experience before and had thought it was all a bunch of
mumbo-jumbo. Now he didn't know what to think or do. The
experience spoke for itself, but it was a bit overwhelming.

Although Paul had several more void experiences, he never
reached the level of intensity he had that first night. However, by
the time he went home his pain was much diminished, and I
recall watching him doing backflips in the swimming pool, when
only a few days earlier, he had been unable to walk down a couple
of steps without wincing in pain.

The best medicine is probably one which not only relieves
symptoms but in the process helps us to rediscover meaning and
leads us back to ourselves again. There was little doubt that, in
Paul's case, the power animal experience had made that vital
connection. He left us keen to get on with his life and determined to return to his home town to search out the traditional
wisdom he had always spurned in the past.

# Chapter 15

# ELECTROCUTION & BURNS

*Love is the unfamiliar Name*
*Behind the hands which wove*
*The intolerable shirt of flame*
*Which human power cannot remove.*
*We only live, only suspire*
*Consumed by either fire or fire.*

— T.S. Eliot

*B*urns and electrocutions can leave scars on the body-mind which go far beyond the visible. Some of our most interesting cases have been people injured by fire and electrical currents. These people often appear perfectly normal but feel far from well and report symptoms and experiences which baffle conventional medicine.

Those who have been electrocuted often struggle with "post-traumatic stress disorder," suffering from phobias, nightmares, terrifying memories, and other symptoms as diverse as stuttering, impotence, memory loss, depression, blurred vision and poor hearing. Some people describe a sense of being "scrambled," find they cannot think clearly, and have the peculiar sensation of electricity still running through their bodies.

Medicine may do a fine job fixing the outward manifestations of burns with sophisticated grafting techniques to replace damaged skin and heal the physical body. But what use is it all if the individual cannot function because of wounds to the body's subtle electromagnetic field, wounds which grieve and confuse the spirit?

Such damage is real and makes perfect sense if we understand that the body holds a kind of energetic "memory" or electromagnetic imprint of the original injury. But as there is rarely objective evidence of any such thing, medicine is left not knowing what, if anything, to do. So, lives are put on hold while patients shuffle from pillar to post, looking for an answer they cannot find.

## HERMAN : ELECTROCUTION AND "SCRAMBLED BRAIN"

Herman was a thirty-five-year-old man who was exposed to fifteen thousand volts of electricity through a metal fence at work. He lost consciousness momentarily and fell to the ground before his colleagues were able to turn the power off. When they reached him, they noticed his eyes and forehead bulging forward very strangely. Herman was treated for third-degree burns on his left hand and thighs. The electrical shock had apparently entered his body through the hand he had been using to hold onto the fence and had passed out through the thighs and knees, leaving multiple burn marks at the entry and exit sites.

Herman's superficial wounds healed well but a deeper and less visible injury had been done. He started to suffer from headaches, nightmares and flashbacks; and when he tried to think, his mind became a jumble of unrelated ideas crowding chaotically one upon another. He was unable to control his thoughts in any way. If he tried to say something, he would forget what he was talking about halfway through his sentence, and was prevented from performing even simple tasks as he would forget what he was doing as he was doing it.

When Herman tried to describe these difficulties to his physicians, he got little in the way of response. Because he looked normal, they reasoned he should return to work and get on with his life. However, with the mental scrambling, Herman was naturally leery of returning to work, feeling he would be a danger to himself and others; and when his complaints were labelled anxiety, he began to wonder if he were going crazy.

Such is often the way in medicine: we attend to the symptoms we recognize and ignore or put aside all else. So Herman was given one tranquillizer, then another, then an antidepressant, then another tranquillizer, in order to suppress his symptoms. But Herman did not want to be tranquillized. He wanted his brain clear. All the tranquillizers did was slow him down: the scrambling continued but as if in slow motion, and a slow scramble was really no better than a fast scramble. No one seemed to understand, and Herman grew more and more depressed and angry at his predicament. He really wanted to pull himself together, but the plain fact was that he couldn't.

ELECTRICAL AFTERSHOCK

Herman was fairly desperate when he came to us. He listened to what we had to offer and determined to give it his best shot. There was nothing to lose.

"It feels just like the electricity is still in my body," Herman admitted to me. "I can feel the tingles, especially in my fingers and in my thighs, and the scrambling in my head just never goes away. I'm so tuned in to electricity I can tell if there is an electrical storm coming — sometimes a couple of days ahead. I get very uncomfortable and my symptoms intensify. I can't go near large electrical power centres either."

From an energetic perspective, a jolt of electricity of the magnitude Herman had encountered would have to leave a large residue in the body-mind. We had seen the energetic consequences of minor car accidents wreak havoc in the body, so what the residue of such an intense electric charge might do was hard to imagine.

"Would you be willing to do something a bit strange?" I asked Herman. "We have had people in the past who have been electrocuted. It's like they still have electricity running in their bodies. We have had some success attaching a wire to the body and draining off the energy into a bucket of water while we do the bodywork and acupuncture."

"I'll try almost anything," said Herman. "I'd even try snake oil if I thought it might help."

Herman entered the void with total commitment and enthusiasm. Within moments of beginning deep breathing he began screaming in pain. We attached a copper wire to his right thigh and led it down into a big bucket of water. Herman's face went a dark red and his eyes seemed to bulge out of his head but he stayed with it.

After it was all over, he fell asleep for three hours, waking to say he felt calmer than he had in eighteen months. Something, he said, had gone out of him. "And I had this remarkable dream," he said as he became more animated. "I don't normally dream very much. In one way the dream was very ordinary but it seemed to be all about what is going on for me and seemed to me to be saying that I'm going to get better. In the dream I was having all kinds of bodywork all at the same time — acupuncture, deep massage, Reiki, and someone was teaching me relaxation techniques. It was really wild. And I felt like I've never felt for years. It's like my body knows it is going to heal."

I had to agree. That dream heralded the beginning of a profound change in Herman. He improved day by day and within a week seemed a completely different person. He entered the void each session, reliving the pain and the intense memories which he had been trying to put out of his mind since his accident, and worked with his feelings and his fear actively. Though we were doing only mild bodywork to encourage the electricity to drain from his legs into the water, Herman's shouts and screams could be heard throughout the building. Something remarkable seemed to be happening and the changes increased by the day.

Then one day Herman had a vision.

"I saw the man," he announced quite matter-of-factly.

"What man?" I asked.

"The man," he said, as if I should know. "He was dressed in white robes, and had a full beard. He stood right in front of me and raised his hands on either side of my head. Then there was a blast of energy like a thunderbolt from his hands and it went through my temples and ran down through my whole body."

Then he started to giggle and then, from somewhere deep in his belly, he laughed. And for the next five days, he laughed and laughed almost uncontrollably. I found I couldn't look at Herman without smiling because he was always chuckling away to himself. It was as if he had deciphered a great cosmic joke.

At first I wondered whether he was having a psychotic break, talking about a man in white robes wandering around the building. But I've learned not to question healing experiences. In any case, my fears were quickly laid to rest because the laughter and healing in Herman were quite genuine. Whether Herman had seen "the man" or not I have no idea. Indeed, just who "the man" was is not entirely clear since Herman never actually put a name to him. But certainly he had seen something which had great meaning and the experience seemed to cement the huge change we'd seen in him.

Toward the end of his stay with us Herman took me aside and said, "You know, my brain is clear for the first time in eighteen months. That drainage procedure with the wire and the bucket of water really does work. Seemed like we were playing Frankenstein there for a moment, but I could feel the electricity coming out of me, big time. And my mind is calm. I can think! You've no idea what it is like to not be able to think! My life has been a complete mess since I was injured and no one has been able to understand what I was going through."

Herman left us saying he felt ninety percent pain free. He was in such high spirits I was concerned he might crash, as people sometimes do; but I also knew we could see him again if it was necessary.

## HELGA : ELECTROCUTION AND DISSOCIATION

Helga was a twenty-nine-year-old woman who had been electrocuted at work when she put her hand into what she thought was a dead electrical socket to fix a broken light switch. It turned out to be very much alive. As is often the case with electrocution victims, she had held onto the wire for some time, unable to let go, before someone had turned off the power, and had been unconscious for several minutes afterwards.

Although Helga seemed to return to normal, she never recovered full function in her right arm, though tests showed there was nothing physically wrong with it. Helga complained that the arm didn't work properly though she could use it quite adequately if asked to. She said she just "couldn't bring herself" to use it regularly. It was an odd phrase to use of one's own body, suggestive of both disgust and intense fear. It was as though she just didn't want to know about the arm.

Her feelings against it were so strong, in fact, she had even requested that it be amputated, something the surgeons had so far refused to do. It was a strange situation, but as the hand was also cold to the touch, I guessed that the imprint of the electric shock might have been sufficient to produce an extreme psychic dissociation.

Helga seemed willing to work on the problem and though she approached acupuncture with a great deal of trepidation, it did not take much for her to reach the edge of the void. Just as she began to pass the breathing barrier, and begin shaking, however, she would turn her head to the left, away from the injured area, and lose consciousness — just as if she were being diverted from her goal by an unseen traffic barrier.

I wondered if Helga had not only psychically disowned her arm but had used to it hold all the electrical residue in order to free the rest of her body for normal functioning. There was little doubt she still had electricity in her body, in much the same way as Herman had. She described similar sensations of a current running in her arm and difficulty with her memory and with concentration.

When Helga realized how she was turning her head away from the injury and interrupting her entry to the void, she asked if I would turn it back at the appropriate moment. But despite her best intentions, she fought me all the way, and her face remained averted from the arm she seemed to so loathe. We seemed to have met an impenetrable barrier.

Next we attached a copper wire to her hand and led it down into a big bucket of water. As she began to enter the void, I dripped water on her face to cool her as she entered the experience of searing heat. Her face went puce. As it did so she screamed and averted her face, turning her head to the left as her arm started to shake uncontrollably. Try as we might, we could not get Helga to look at her arm. She seemed unable to move, as if paralysed, except for this vibrating arm and she began shouting, "Get rid of it! Cut it off!"

The meaning of her head turning adamantly away from the injured arm every time it "came alive" as she neared the void became clear. It was as if the body-mind absolutely refused to admit the insult that had been done to it. At some very deep level she had rejected her arm altogether.

Despite much effort, Helga's struggle to accept her arm progressed slowly. Whenever she entered the void, she seemed to hit a wall of terror and pain which she was unable to penetrate.

That point may have represented the terror of the memory and her reluctance to enter and relive it.

As of this writing, Helga is far from better, and is beginning to develop cataracts. Since cataracts are most unusual in someone so young, I am tempted to think that although there is no way of knowing for sure, there might be some relation between the electrical shock and their development. In other words, the electrical energy in her body might be slowly "cooking" her lenses, as heat cooks and clouds the white of an egg.

## LUIGI : METHYLENE BURNS

Luigi was an Italian immigrant who worked in a chemical plant for several years after coming to Canada in 1976. He was badly burned one day when an explosion occurred on a nearby workbench in the lab. Luigi was a tall, imposing man with rugged features who must have created quite a stir in his day. The injury had involved much of his face: the area round the mouth, his nose, and both ears were scarred, but the rugged good looks could still be guessed through the skin grafts.

But despite extensive reconstructive surgery, the evidence of injury was hard to hide. His ears were misshapen, his mouth pulled down to the right, and his nose was angulated. It took a few minutes to get past his deformities on first meeting him but as I got to know him I hardly noticed his scarring.

The same could not be said for Luigi. He had never been able to accept the face he saw in the mirror every day. He felt his life was forever changed and he had become increasingly withdrawn, even hermetic, refusing to see his friends or engage in social activity. And, slowly but surely, the vicious cycle of increasing isolation, depression and irritability made him unpleasant to be around.

## POST-EXPLOSION AMNESIA

Luigi recalled the explosion but had no memory of the moments immediately afterward. Methylene burns with a cold flame invisible to the eye so at the time his arms were on fire he could feel burning but see nothing — a peculiar contradiction of perception by experience which he felt may have contributed to his loss of memory.

He recalled the ambulance ride to hospital, too, but did not understand — until sometime later — how extensive his injuries were. Yet all these areas had been repaired by skin grafts, and apart from the scarring on his face, there seemed little reason why Luigi could not get on with his life. He was physically able, was not in any great physical pain, so what was stopping him?

The answer lay in the dimension of mind and spirit. Like other burn victims, Luigi was severely handicapped by something that was invisible to others. Every day was an agony. He dreaded facing himself in the mirror, and loathed the ritual of skin care — putting cream on the exposed areas and applying bandages. He suffered, too, from the constant reminder of his injury as the stubble of his beard irritated the grafts.

Then there were the mental obsessions. Luigi kept replaying the accident over and over in his mind like a broken record. "If only I had done this, or that, perhaps it would never have happened." But worse than that he couldn't actually complete the terrible memory, which would reach a certain point and then stop and go back to the beginning. He couldn't get his mind around what had actually happened; and his mind seemed bent on repeating the experience in the hopes of breaking through the barrier. But the completed memory never came. The broken record continued to play the same events, over and over, and nothing new ever came to consciousness. No wonder he was getting depressed.

"Why do you want to know?" I asked him one day. "I mean, what difference does it really make now?"

"I don't know," Luigi told me "I really don't. But there is something there that I need."

Luigi entered the void like a man with a mission, putting every ounce of himself into a superhuman effort to retrieve memories. I wondered whether this mission was wise but did nothing to discourage him, always reminding myself when I think to interfere with someone's path, that each of us accomplishes our own healing the only way we know how. Interference from outside just gets in the way, and projects others' expectations onto the process.

On entering the void, Luigi's body shook for a half an hour until he was soaking with sweat and totally exhausted.

"Perhaps you are trying too hard," I suggested eventually.

"What else can I do?" he asked, wondering how anything could be achieved without effort.

"Too much effort can be as unrewarding as too little," I said, realizing it was an inadequate answer, but nothing else came to mind.

Something must have got through to him, however, because the next time he came, Luigi was definitely more relaxed. He entered the void gently and after several minutes of shaking and breathing, he seemed to go into another realm.

The next thing I knew he was shouting, "My arms are on fire! I'm burning! I'm burning!" His hands were vibrating rapidly and he was looking from one to the other and back again. We got several cool damp towels and draped them over his arms.

"You're safe," I reassured him. "It's just a memory. You've got cool cloths on your arms and legs now, just keep going, stay with it." The suggestion seemed to help and he was able to go on. After it was over, he recounted his experience to us.

"It was really weird," he said. "It was just like I was back there at the fire. I could feel my arms burning even though I couldn't see any flames. That's what happened you know, that methylene burned cold, without a flame you could see."

"Yes, I know. But how come only your arms and face were burned, Luigi?" I asked him.

"The rest of my body was protected by an old pair of overalls I was wearing. They got pretty badly burned but they protected me, thank goodness, or things would have been much worse."

Strangely, it turned out that the old overalls were still around. "You know I never threw them away," Luigi admitted to me. "They are still down in the basement in a plastic bag."

"Why?" I asked innocently.

"I haven't been able to look at those overalls since the explosion," he said. "Just the thought of them freaks me out. But for some reason I want to keep them too. I can't get rid of them. Perhaps I want to be reminded — I don't know. I asked my partner to put them away three years ago, and she did, and they've been down in our basement ever since. I can't bring myself to get rid of the bag, or even to look at it."

Perhaps here, I thought, was the container of memories Luigi was looking for. In any case, no harm could come from confronting and exploring this fear. I gently suggested to Luigi that if he was willing to bring the overalls in, we could help him explore the intense feelings their presence might engender.

"I'm not sure I could do that," he said, looking absolutely terrified. "I'm so frightened by them I haven't been able to take them out of the bag for three years. In fact, I get terrified just thinking about them."

It took several days of gentle encouragement but eventually Luigi found the courage. He appeared one day carrying a small plastic garbage bag and dropped it on the floor of the room.

"You've no idea what it took for me to bring this in," he said looking shaken. "I'm not sure how I made it here at all."

"Why don't you take them out of the bag and put them on?" I got right to the point.

"I couldn't possibly!" he blurted.

Part of me couldn't believe this exchange. How could anyone be scared of a pair of pants? But Luigi was obviously terrified.

"Come on," I said. "Look, we're right here so if anything bad happens we'll be with you. If you take some deep breaths as you open the bag you'll be able to enter the void immediately and we may discover something. We'll be right here with you," I reassured him.

He looked at me for a long moment, then, remarkably, went straight over to the bag and picked it up off the floor where he'd dropped it. Though his hands were shaking so much he almost dropped it again, he managed to open it slowly and, after some hesitation, reached inside. He grasped the old overalls which had not seen the light of day for three years and pulled them out. He seemed alright so I pressed him further.

"Okay Luigi, why don't you put them on?" Again he recoiled.

"Nothing bad has happened so far," I reasoned; but he was extremely reluctant to go any further. A few more minutes of gentle persuasion eventually did the trick. Luigi dropped the pant legs to the floor and began to pull them on, one leg at a time. Suddenly, he started to laugh.

This was the last thing I expected. Shouting, yes; crying, yes; but laughter had me completely flummoxed. I said nothing and just waited.

"I don't believe it!" Luigi called out, his face dazed and elated at once. "These *aren't the overalls!* I mean, they're not the overalls I was wearing when I got burned! It's another pair.

How extraordinary — to think that for three years I've been scared of a plastic bag in the basement with a perfectly ordinary pair of old overalls in it!" Luigi started to laugh again and his laughter grew heartier by the minute as it seemed to swell inside of him.

"Boy, that's really something, that is! Who would have thought? What a bunch of nonsense I've been getting into!" he roared. "That really takes the biscuit. You know, I always thought the overalls were jinxed but really I'm jinxed, or I've jinxed myself, one of the two."

I couldn't help but join Luigi in his amazement, not only because of what he said, but also because the situation had demonstrated beautifully the nature of the problem he was facing. No one could have told him this thing: he'd have denied it. But the experience spoke for itself. We watched as Luigi's armouring fell away and he began to rediscover the man he used to be. A door was opened in his psyche and he became keen to explore the inner man.

FLASHBACK

It so often seems that people heal in spite of what we do, not because of it. Situations arise when we are open which can generate a healing crisis. Luigi's experience with his overalls was another example of a catalyst at work.

On another occasion, Luigi entered the void and reached the now familiar place where his forearms were burning. We placed the cool towels over his arms again and encouraged him to go deeper into the experience.

"I'm burning! I'm burning!" he kept repeating. "I've got to get out of here." He started scuffling and stumbling as if he was trying to find his way about. Then his legs kicked as if he was jumping and he shouted, "Someone get me out of here! Where is the door...the door!" More scuffling followed, then Luigi collapsed in a heap. His shoulders shook violently as great sobs burst forth and his eyes flickered back and forth with the tell-tale signs of inner visions. He lay there for ten or fifteen minutes crying quietly.

"You know," he said, when he recovered and was ready to talk, "I never thought I would ever find out what happened. But just now I saw the accident all over again — the whole thing — from start to finish. In the past, after I felt my arms burning, I would kind of go blank and everything would become a blur until I came around in the ambulance."

"But this time it was different. I guess after the overalls incident I feel different — not so scared of everything. Something changed inside. I was totally calm and I could see the whole thing. I got up off the floor, moved a big, heavy cabinet which had crashed down in front of me, and found the doorway before collapsing in the hall outside the room. I was only there for about fifteen seconds before someone came and picked me up and carried me outside."

Then he said the thing which indicated the depth of his healing: "You know, there was nothing else I could have done under the circumstances."

Luigi's demeanour had changed. His concerns with his appearance seemed to shift as well after this session and he began to engage the other participants in active and lively dialogue. Gone was his anxiety and inner turmoil, and in its place was a calmness which rubbed off on everyone around.

Luigi returned to his life with a renewed enthusiasm and a determination to get on with his life's work. He visited us at the clinic a year later. He was busy running his farm and had married the woman he had lived with for the past five years. He seemed to move away from his obsession with the accident to engage the world from a different place.

## Chapter 16

# HEART TROUBLE

*A merry heart maketh*
*a cheerful countenance;*
*but a sorrow of the heart*
*the spirit is broken.*

— Proverbs 15:13

*K*ieran was a small, slight 42-year-old woman with a
pale complexion and chronic exhaustion. A full head of flaming
red hair stood out in stark contrast to her morbid pallor, as if
pointing to more exuberant possibilities in her character. But for
now, any such possibilities lay dormant. She had been in great
difficulty for several years, following quadruple bypass surgery for
a massive heart attack, and was so tired most of the time that she
could hardly walk across a room without getting short of breath.

Kieran had blurred memories of the whole experience. The
only thing she remembered clearly was the trip in the ambulance; after that, things were pretty much blank. She couldn't
recall much of her hospital stay, and after her surgery, which was
declared a success, she remained a "cardiac cripple," with very
little tolerance for activity. Her heart could not tolerate any
physical stress, and she often became short of breath as her heart
failed to meet the needs of the moment. When her heart "failed"
in this way, the poor pumping action meant that fluids backed
up into her lungs, and she became breathless. She took a number of drugs to counteract the situation: digoxin, to improve her
heart's function, a diuretic to remove excess fluid from the
lungs, and something else to reduce the peripheral arterial resistance. But the medications were frequently inadequate and

when fluid built up too much, she would visit the nearest emergency department for intravenous therapy to clear it.

That Kieran should have had a heart attack so young was probably due to a combination of her genetic make-up and a few unhealthy habits. She had a family history of high cholesterol and several other family members had had early heart attacks. She also smoked excessively. Although she was aware that smoking was particularly hazardous for her given her family history, she was still smoking a pack a day when she came to see us.

It's mystifying that people will continue self-destructive habits even after they have suffered extremely unpleasant consequences. I'll never forget an old patient whom I saw as a fledgling medical student. Like Kieran, he had cardiovascular disease. The old fellow had lost all his fingers and toes, one by one, to compromised circulation, until he had only two fingers left, the index and little fingers of his left hand. Even so, he continued to smoke, holding his cigarette precariously between these two remaining fingers. The picture of him sitting in the hallway, enjoying what he felt was his last remaining pleasure, left a lasting impression.

Surprisingly perhaps, Kieran's heart trouble was not her primary concern. Instead she complained of severe, unremitting pain in her right foot, which was so sore she could hardly put any weight on it. Surgery had unfortunately left her with some nerve damage — a peroneal nerve palsy — in her foot which had resulted in a foot drop and constant pain in the sole of her foot. But besides that, the circulation in her feet was no great shakes. She had arterial pulses, indicating the large vessel circulation was okay, but the skin on her legs and arms had the blotchy appearance typical of someone whose small vessel circulation was compromised. Slight pressure on the skin produced blanching which lasted for several minutes.

It was apparent that the medical system had done all it could for Kieran, and then left her to get on with her life. But now that she was on her own, she felt completely abandoned. Her physicians could monitor her drugs, treat her heart failure when necessary and berate her for her refusal to quit smoking. But they could do nothing to help Kieran's spirit which had taken a terrible beating.

Years went by. Eventually, Kieran realized it was time to do something different. Her life was deeply unsatisfying; and with a remarkable calm determination and sense of responsibility for herself which I have rarely seen in others, she set out to heal.

From the moment we met, it was clear she was ready. While she was very anxious about what might be required of her, she had essentially given up looking for someone else to blame for her misfortunes, and arrived at our centre ready to explore and learn. I could not have asked for a better attitude in a client, and in spite of my own fears and misgivings around working with someone with such severe heart disease, I looked forward to the challenge of sharing her journey.

At first, Kieran said that it would be hard for her to let anyone touch her foot, it was so painful; but it wasn't long before she decided to let us work with it anyway. It seemed that once she acknowledged her fear, she was able to face it and get on with the exploration. It was a characteristic I saw several times over the ten days she was with us.

During her first session, after she had been lying down breathing fairly deeply for a few moments, I touched her foot very gently. Almost immediately her shoulders jumped forward quite violently and flopped back. I pulled away, but she didn't seem terribly shaken, so I gingerly touched the area again, and the same thing happened. Her body was speaking in a curious way but it was pretty clear what it was trying to convey and the many years I have spent in hospitals allowed me to understand her body language.

Most hospitals have a cardiac arrest team who stimulate the heart electrically by placing paddles directly over it and administering a shock. Kieran's body seemed to be imitating the movements typical of this kind of cardiac resuscitation. While Kieran couldn't remember if she had had this treatment, it seemed quite likely that she had. The "cardiac arrest cart" is a fixture in emergency wards, and paddles are available in most ambulances. Patients who have collapsed and who arrive in a busy emergency department may have the paddles applied whether they need them or not.

An electrical shock is an electrical shock no matter where it comes from, and there will be residue in the body-mind as with any other kind of electrocution. It seemed likely to me that there would be after-effects in Kieran similar to those we had seen in other survivors of electric shock.

At our next session, Kieran said she was surprised by the ease with which she had tolerated our manipulations of her foot and was willing to let us explore her pain a little further. I hooked a wire up to her foot and drained it into a big bucket of water — just as I had done with other clients suffering from electrical injury — and placed my finger on the tender point on her foot. This time, the flopping movements increased, Kieran's eyes nearly closed, and she seemed to go to the edge of an altered state of consciousness. Her eyes flickered rapidly, reflecting intense inner experience and her attention seemed to turn inward.

Suddenly, Kieran got frightened and started to wheeze. Gasping for breath and clutching at her chest and throat, she started to inch her way across the floor as if she was trying to crawl away from something or someone, all the while exclaiming, "It's hot! It's hot! It's hot!" Since the bucket of water was handy, we drenched a towel and put it around her neck and upper chest, telling her she was totally safe and that what she was experiencing was just a memory.

As I reassured her, the fear drained from her face and she began to breathe more normally. Meanwhile, her body shook and vibrated as if she were having an epileptic seizure. This went on for several minutes, then she gradually settled down and breathed more easily. But it was two hours before she stopped shaking.

The following morning, Kieran had an episode of breathlessness due to a fluid buildup in her chest and had to go to the hospital for a diuretic injection. Since the void experience had been quite frightening for her, I was pleased to see Kieran return a couple of hours later, keen to continue the work she had begun. We talked about the incident to help her to put the whole thing in perspective. There was little doubt she was quite shaken by her first encounter with the void and I would not have been surprised if she had been reluctant to go back.

"Do you think the acupuncture had anything to do with the water in my lungs?" she asked. "It scared the daylights out of me."

"Yes and no," I relied cryptically. "You've had attacks of pulmonary oedema from time to time, so you might have been due for one anyway. On the other hand, it's perfectly possible that your fear could focus in the cardiovascular system, increase peripheral resistance and put more load on the heart. So the build-up of fluids could have been a result of your fear of the experience, even though it wasn't caused by the experience itself."

"The decision you have to make now," I told her, "is whether you are willing to explore this fear more deeply, even though your first experience was so terrifying to you. All I can say is the second time in will likely be a bit easier, and we'll anticipate things better, too, and be right there with you."

This left Kieran in a quandary. She wanted to do what was necessary to heal but she was not sure she wanted to face her terror again, especially now she knew it could land her in hospital. We spent a lot of time talking through her fears and helping her get enough courage together to face the unknown with a measure of calmness and trust.

Kieran took up the challenge. At the start of the next session I hooked her foot up to the wire again and gently touched the sole. She took a couple of deep breaths and within moments started to shake all over in her now-familiar "cardiac resuscitation" flop-and-jerk style. She seemed to have come to terms with her fear and was psyched up to experience the void without resistance. There was no wheezing and no terror, and Kieran proceeded to shake and tremble in an altered state of consciousness for forty-five minutes. During that time she went far into the void and became unavailable to ordinary conversation. When eventually she did come back to the rational world, her hands were warm for the first time in five years and her mottled skin had cleared. Her transformation amazed us all, and she retained some conscious memory of her experiences to boot.

Kieran told us she had relived her hospital experience, saw the emergency department, the doctors and nurses looking down at her, trying to save her life. She saw the cardiac paddles and the operating room, and re-experienced going under anaesthetic, all of which had been blotted from her mind. She seemed surreally calm, completely different from the woman who first came to us.

But these changes were just the beginning. Next, a very curious thing happened: Kieran lost her hearing. She had had no problem with her ears in the past but now she said she couldn't hear people talking to her, as if there were a constant background buzz obscuring her senses.

"You'll have to speak up," she said when we began talking the next day. "I can't seem to hear anything today."

It was a bit puzzling. Kieran had never had trouble with her hearing and my first impulse was to check for wax in her ear canals or an infection. But somehow I intuited that something else was happening. I resisted the urge to medicalize the situation and instead trusted my hunch.

Perhaps Kieran was just having difficulty absorbing and integrating her new experiences. Things had been a little overwhelming, to say the least. Given the intensity of her experiences in the void, I felt sure the problem was a metaphorical representation of an extreme attention to the chaos of her changing inner life. Kieran was penetrating her inner defences for the first time and intuiting a deeper truth for her life. What she really needed to hear were the feelings and promptings of her own heart.

That interpretation suggested the acupuncture point "Tinggong," or "Palace of hearing," which directly addresses this issue. So at the next session, while Kieran once again breathed her way toward the void, I put a needle at that spot. A moment or two later, the familiar flopping indicated she had reached her goal, and she continued to shake effortlessly for about twenty minutes. I waited to see what would happen.

That night Kieran had a very vivid dream. It seemed ordinary enough but clearly had great meaning for her.

"I don't normally dream at all," she said. "And even if I had had a dream, it wouldn't occur to me to pay any attention to it."

"What was it about?" I asked.

"Well I was in my living room, arguing with my son about keeping his room clean. He's totally chaotic ... you know ... never cleans up after himself, and his room's an unbelievable pig-stye. I just don't know what to do with him most of the time. We're always fighting about it. Well this time, you know ... in the dream, that is ... after the usual threats and insults, he stopped to think for a moment, then offered to clean up the whole house. Then he went ahead and did it ... cleaned up the whole house ... completely spick and span. I know it seems silly but he would just never do that. It was totally out of character. He just completely changed, right in front of my eyes. ... The funny thing is ... I think it must be me who's changed."

Kieran had said it all. The dream was remarkable. Mundane as it seemed, she felt the dream was speaking directly to her experience in the void, and a curiosity arose in her which changed her view of the world for ever. Things which before seemed random and disconnected were now connected in such a way as to make a profound difference to her life. She began to intuit meaning in her symptoms and began to guess at the deeper meaning her heart disease might hold.

The pain in Kieran's foot was greatly diminished by the end of the program, and she had begun to recognize how it served her as a doorway to new realizations. Her attitude toward her life was totally transformed. She wondered whether her heart disease was a reflection of her inability to listen to her heart's desires and resolved to be more attentive.

That resolution led to deeper questions. What were those dreams which she had never fulfilled? What did she really want to do with her life? Ironically, Kieran felt she had put off questions such as these in the past because her heart disease was "in the way." Now, for the first time, she considered the possibility that her heart disease might be the result of her heart's dis-ease.

## EPILOGUE

I saw Kieran about a year later. Her foot pain was very much better and she had had only one episode of heart failure, and that she attributed to stress she had handled badly. The foot drop and peroneal palsy remained but that was to be expected. Her skin tone was also much improved, the mottling of her skin and the cold extremities were gone. Her demeanour, however, was most impressive. No longer chronically fatigued and depressed, she had started a small handicrafts business and was seriously thinking of terminating her disability pension.

# Chapter 17

# KIDNEY TROUBLE

*... medicine is going more and more in the direction of high tech for evaluation and diagnosis when people are crying out for someone who cares for them, someone who will sit down and actually listen to them.*

— David Felten M.D., Ph.D.

*L*orna was a twenty-six-year-old woman who was first diagnosed with renal disease as a child of six. Since then, her kidney function had deteriorated until, at thirty, she had needed a kidney transplant. The operation had resulted in drug reactions, a urinary obstruction requiring further surgery, and chronic rejection of the grafted kidney, leading to kidney failure.

While waiting for another organ to become available, Lorna was prescribed a number of drugs, including cyclosporin, prednisone, and azathioprine to suppress her immune response, and vasodilators to promote blood supply to the ailing kidney. So far, she had avoided dialysis, but it was a distinct possibility she would need it soon — a prospect which she found quite terrifying.

If Lorna's doctors were puzzled by the rejection, they did not show it. Scientific medicine tends to volunteer statistics as an explanation of the disease process, and views organ rejection as "just something that happens" with a certain frequency in transplant surgery. Seeking deeper explanations is generally regarded by the medical profession as futile, if not plain fanciful.

However for Lorna, the impersonal statistical explanation was insufficient. After all, having barely surfaced as an adult, she was facing multiple surgeries with no guarantees. In fact, with her track record, it was quite likely her body would also reject further transplants. And each rejected transplant would take her one step nearer dialysis and an early death. Her mortality loomed close and made her desperate.

For some time, Lorna had wanted to explore alternatives. Her physicians, however, were unsupportive and actively discouraged her — in spite of her poor response to drug treatment — pointing out that her life was in the balance and that unproven therapies might jeopardize her health. In the end, their strictures only made her hostile and increasingly suspicious that the physicians were more concerned with their transplant program than they were with her health. She began to hold them responsible for everything that was not going well — the transplant rejection, the drug toxicity, and the surgical complications; and she decided she wanted no more treatment from them.

Lorna's first idea was to change physicians, but it proved to be a frustrating exercise, as might have been predicted. When we are chronically ill, changing physicians may not solve the problem, in part because the new relationship can simply replicate the old. Scientific medicine has standardized its treatment regimens to such a degree that there is often very little variation in treatment from physician to physician. A transplant is a transplant; and cyclosporin and prednisone are the same wherever you get them. Furthermore, doctors are naturally put on their guard when seeing patients who complain about their previous physicians. So, we may find our new physician even more guarded than our old while we are recommended precisely the same treatment regimen. In these circumstances, our rage has nowhere to go, and the fact that we really do have a choice of treatments — since all treatments are voluntary — is lost in an atmosphere of control and resentment against the establishment.

## EXPLORING UNRELATED PAIN

Not knowing where else to turn, Lorna eventually found her way to our clinic. As it happened, she was also suffering from leg pain from an old tibial fracture sustained in a car accident, and she thought perhaps a holistic approach might allow her to deal more effectively with the stress and pain she was facing. It was a long shot — but she knew she had to do something different, or else resign herself to her deteriorating health.

When Lorna arrived, she was distrusting, angry, frustrated and hostile. She had no reason to trust us any more than anyone else she had dealt with, except that we did offer a different approach, and one which did not rely on drugs and surgery. In her view, that was one small factor in our favour.

I was initially struck by Lorna's appearance. She had a bulky physique and extraordinarily tight hips. Her thighs, arms and torso were so thick and her hips so tight that she couldn't pull her legs apart and her gait was unnatural. When she walked, her legs seemed to move around each other as though they were in each other's way; and her strangely immobile pelvis made her look as though she were wrapped in a straitjacket from her neck to her ankles.

Not surprisingly, perhaps, Lorna was initially very frightened of bodywork and acupuncture. It took her several days of settling in before she took her first tentative steps. We knew that her reticence signalled that trust was a major issue so we didn't push her but waited for her to initiate her own process. Meanwhile, we explained the mechanics of guided hyperventilation, the concept of the void, and described common experiences during bodywork, and told her she was free to stop at any time. Mostly we just focused on creating rapport and trust.

Then one day, Lorna announced she was ready. She dove in with enthusiasm, using her unusual physical strength to push her hyperventilation to the limit; and within moments, we had a major struggle on our hands. After only a few deep breaths, she began to lash out, kicking and screaming, and beating anyone who came close with her fists.

Then, without warning, she began to shout. "Get off me ... get away ... you son of a bitch!" Then at the top of her lungs she screamed, "Get the fuck off me, you bastard!"

I backed away, thinking for a moment she really was talking to me. "Do you want me to stop, Lorna? Or are you just talking to ... whoever?" I asked, genuinely concerned the situation might be getting out of hand.

"No, not you, for heaven's sake ... I'm not talking to you," she reassured me, signalling me to carry on. "You told me I could say whatever I wanted ... so I am."

I felt relieved for the moment. Clearly, Lorna didn't want to stop at all. Far from it, in a way she was just getting started. She had heard my initial instruction to say "stop" if she wanted me to stop, and so her outburst was simply the expression of a something she had stored for some time. And sure enough, as soon as we started bodywork again, she continued her diatribe.

"Get off. Don't come near me. Leave me alone! Get the fuck off me! Fuck *off*!" she yelled, kicking and lashing out all around, making it difficult to get anywhere near her, let alone do any bodywork. The more I tried to work with her, the more she fought me off — not as if to stop the process, but rather because to fight is what her body seemed to want. She was as strong as an ox and she plainly enjoyed the scrap.

After that first session Lorna's hands, which were chronically cold, warmed up for the first time in years, and she felt more relaxed than she had in a very long time. However, I was more than a bit uncomfortable with the process. Lorna's body seemed to be responding to a perceived threat. Since there was nothing actually threatening her in the moment, we were clearly dealing with a remembered menace; and it seemed no ordinary memory of an accident or physical trauma. I had the distinct feeling I knew where Lorna was going to go next. Everything pointed to physical or sexual trauma of some kind.

The tight hips, the tight pelvis, the awkward gait, the fighting and the kidney failure — it all pointed to an energy block in the lower back and pelvis, something which by now we were thoroughly familiar with from other clients. But no matter how often I see it, the surfacing of such violent memories remains disturbing.

Meanwhile we wondered whether her childhood experience was connected to her kidney failure and whether the tension in her body had been sufficient to damage her organs. And indeed, whether we would ever find out. Bodywork by definition requires contact, but it didn't look as if we were going to get close enough to do any significant hands-on work.

So we had to come up with an alternative, a way to work safely with Lorna, to explore the tight pelvic musculature, while simultaneously respecting her body's natural desire to fight.

"These sessions are proving a tad difficult," I said, making a deliberate understatement in the hopes of finding a nice way of putting things. "We don't seem to be able to get close enough to you to actually explore any tension patterns, so I don't think we are getting anywhere very fast. We really need to begin working with your tight thighs and pelvis, but it's tough to get close enough for some contact. Could you back off sufficiently to let me at least do a bit of acupressure on the thighs. Is it that you don't feel safe yet? ... because remember, you can always stop at any time if you want to." I repeated the instruction to be absolutely sure she understood.

"I know that," she answered sincerely. "No ... that's not the problem ... I feel totally safe with you guys. It's just me ... I feel so pissed off I want to scream at anyone and everyone, especially if anyone even thinks of coming close. ... I've had it up to here with doctor's examinations, endless blood tests and so on ... so I'm shouting it out. Don't worry — it's not you," she said as if to reassure me again.

"Thanks," I acknowledged her. "That's a relief ... but I think if we want to go forward from here, you are going to have to allow some contact. How about if you let me a bit closer, then let each session lead exactly where it wants to go, knowing that you are free to stop whenever.

"No problem," she agreed. "Let's give it a go. I think I'm ready ... you know ... I'm sure you know ... I'm really just afraid of myself, and what I might find if I were really to let go."

With those words, Lorna put her finger right on the real issue — which really we all face, which is what we might find if we were to totally surrender, not to someone or something else, but to *ourselves*. In so doing, Lorna demonstrated her intuitive understanding of the depth of her inner rage.

She went on. "That first experience — you know, when I was able to shout at the top of my lungs — was so positive, so powerful for me that, really, I'm ready to do what it takes to get to the bottom of this thing."

So we went on. We began working with Lorna's thighs as much as we could, trying to push them apart and ease the tightness. However, Lorna was immensely strong and several sessions of intense wrestling ensued, much like the first sessions, which left us no farther ahead in our efforts to open her pelvis. No doubt as a child she had been vulnerable but as an adult it was hard to imagine anyone physically abusing her, she was so strong. And yet despite it all, her adult strength could do nothing to mitigate the feeling of vulnerability which lay at the core of her being, and her need to defend herself at every moment of her life. Lorna seemed ruled by memory, her immense physical armouring the mark of a woman literally hobbled by old terrors.

From here on it is hard to even describe what happened. In such dynamic encounters, the unknown remains unknown in each moment, and it is not always clear what is happening, or even why. We just have to go with whatever is given us, moment by moment. Battle succeeded battle, and it seemed that we were getting nowhere but something was certainly shifting in Lorna. Trust seemed to be flooding back into her as if it were a physical substance and by the end of the program, she seemed a completely different person.

We knew that her chronic muscular tension, as far as we could measure it by biofeedback, had been reduced dramatically. But more striking was the complete evaporation of the hostility she had showed us. In its place was an exuberant playfulness and a joyful enthusiasm.

It remained to be seen whether there would be any change in her kidneys however, so we were elated two months later when Lorna contacted us to say that her kidney deterioration had stabilized and indeed, had actually improved sufficiently for her to be taken off the critical list for a repeat transplant. Lorna's physicians were mystified at her improvement but apparently not mystified enough to question her about what she had been doing. They simply assumed that the drug therapy they had prescribed was finally doing the trick. A year later, her improvement was sustained.

PAST AND PRESENT

Lorna's case illustrates the power of the exploratory approach, of even seemingly unrelated problems. As it turned out, her chronic pelvic tension was deeply related to her kidney failure, and the absence of this understanding was seriously compromising her health. Extrapolating from her experience, we might realize the potential significance of all past experiences, which by being a part of our overall gestalt may be contributing to any present problem. That way, we could understand the past being very much here with us in the present.

The idea of past, present and even future, all being *here now* is very much a part of holistic thinking. Indeed, such thinking might be better understood by dispensing with the notion of linear time altogether, and replacing it with the concept of an ever-present moment. Linear time, after all, is just an intellectual construct, just a way of thinking which is useful in so far as it helps us to make appointments, or schedule work.

However, when it comes to the healing journey, a different view of time can be very useful. If we so choose, we can understand our whole history, including everything which we have ever experienced, to be present with us now in the form of memory. Such a perspective eliminates the need to look for discrete causes for why we are ill, and gives us complete freedom to explore the inner world for answers.

No doubt Lorna's kidney transplant was necessary; it just wasn't the whole story. She was also very angry, had been so for a long time, and had no way of letting it out. Her anger was stored in her body waiting to be discovered. Such anger may have had its origin in some childhood experience, some instance of sexual abuse, or may have been something she was born with. But the origin of a feeling is simply not as important as the fact of its presence.

Lorna's exploration of the void allowed her to experience quickly and directly why she was ill, and empowered her to do something about it, all in a relatively short period of time. In so doing, she freed herself from an existence tethered to the medical system, and found a much more normal life.

EPILOGUE

I ran into Lorna two years later at a weekend lecture. She was looking well and happy and told me that her kidneys were still functioning well. There was no more talk of a transplant and she was excited about her life and her future. She had returned to school to fulfil a long-held dream of becoming a teacher.

# Chapter 18

## PHANTOM PAIN

*The greatest thing in the world is for a man to know how to be himself.*

— Montaigne

So-called "phantom pain" refers to the phenomenon of pain felt in a part of the body which no longer exists: when an arm has been amputated and the hand still hurts; when there is pain in the foot but the leg is not there.

When I did ward rounds in the hospital as a medical student years ago I remember encountering phantom pain for the first time. The patient, an elderly man with peripheral vascular disease from diabetes, had had his leg amputated when the circulation to his foot became compromised. The old man, who spoke no English, simply pointed insistently to the place where his foot used to be, indicating that it hurt. I remember absorbing the standard explanation of the phenomenon — that the pain was due to stimulation of the nerve stumps by scar tissue at the stump site — without question, even if it wasn't entirely satisfactory, and seemed to be lacking something I couldn't put my finger on.

A few years later, I learned about Kirlian photography, a technique which records the electromagnetic or energetic field of physical structures on film. When amputated limbs or torn leaves, for example, are photographed using this procedure, the precise shape of the original limb or leaf is revealed in the photograph.

It is as though the objects' energy fields contain a perfect and detailed memory of their original physical structures. Since the advent of this photography, it has been well established that there is an electromagnetic field around physical bodies which approximates the shape of the physical structure of the body but is not limited to it. More fascinating still, this energetic body cannot be amputated: somehow the memory of the original structure remains and can even be photographed. The presence of such a field seems to imply the existence of a refined, and less-than-material matrix upon which physical structure is projected.

Rupert Sheldrake's theory of formative causation may have something to offer on this subject. In *A New Science of Life,* he posits that for all natural forms or complexes there is a pre-existing "morphogenetic" field based on that form's collective memory. This morphogenetic field produces an energetic focus around which a specific physical body precipitates. According to Sheldrake, a giraffe has the form of a giraffe because the giraffe form is held in the collective memory field of generations of giraffes. This theory implies not only a non-material substrate upon which the material body is projected but also that this substrate represents a species' specific memory of previous forms, like a kind of cultural habit.

Sheldrake's field theory challenges the standard mechanistic view of conventional biology and scientific medicine. Further, there is now overwhelming evidence that such energy fields underlie all of what we consider our physical reality. Certainly his theories better explain many puzzling phenomena. In my view, the morphogenetic field he proposes may be similar to the body's electromagnetic field, although less material. While the electromagnetic field is material and measurable, however, Sheldrake implies that the morphogenetic field is "non-material."

## ROGER : PHANTOM ARM PAIN

Despite the awe I'd felt on seeing the luminous and perfect ghostly completion of a torn leaf's "missing" half in Kirlian photographs, the arguments for and against the existence of energetic

fields were largely theoretical speculation in my mind, far removed from the practicalities of everyday medicine, until the
day I met Roger. Roger's left arm had been amputated after it
was crushed by several hundred pounds of falling steel in an
industrial accident, and he had lived since then with unremitting pain in an arm which to the casual observer no longer
existed.

Roger's awareness of his phantom arm was by no means
vague. Besides an unusual coldness in the stump, his very particular sense was that his hand, with the fingers curled up into a
fist, was constantly being crushed in a vice. The only time he
noticed a change was just as he was falling off to sleep, when the
spectral fingers seemed to relax momentarily.

Naturally, conventional medicine had no way to approach
this problem. How could it? If one assumes a strictly structural,
mechanistic body, pain can only be understood where there is
palpable flesh through which nerves can transmit information.
So Roger had come to our program to explore his chronic pain.

When I first described the theory of energy medicine to
Roger, he understood almost immediately because he was living
its precepts. In fact, the more I thought about phantom limb
pain in this context, the more sense it made to me too. After all,
if pain is understood as a stagnation of energy flow in the body,
and that body's energy field is understood to extend beyond the
visible and physical limits we associate with objects, then not
only is there a reason for phantom limb pain to exist but there is
also the possibility of effective treatment. Theoretically, phantom limb pain should respond to the same sort of exploration we
were accustomed to using to understand other physical ills.

The standard explanation of phantom pain is not entirely
wrong. It's just not very useful and doesn't really help people in
pain — largely because it's incomplete. Why, for instance, does
phantom pain relate to the original injury and not the injury of

the amputation? Why did the crushing pain of Roger's original injury continue without reference to the pain — albeit masked — of amputation? The mechanistic explanation is difficult to fathom and leaves too many questions unanswered, whereas the theory of an energy body validates patients' lived experience and gives a solid foundation for understanding the emotional and bodily memory of the trauma.

## THE IMPACT ON SELF-IMAGE

Roger had fought hard to keep going and was working full time helping other injured workers. By turning his disability into an opportunity, he seemed to have found a fulfilling and creative way of life. But his pain continued to harass him, interfering with his daily activities and his sleep, constantly reminding him of the accident and leaving him drained. Despite his great will and determination, he had eventually lost his *joie de vivre* and had become cynical and self-absorbed. His amputation embarrassed him and he hid it whenever he could. He wore his prosthesis even though it was uncomfortable and pulled his sleeve down as far as it would go, hoping no one would notice. He felt that people were constantly looking at him and he felt unacceptable — even less than human — without both his arms.

"Why do you feel that way?" I asked him one day. "You know, when we first met I didn't even notice your arm, your prosthetic is so good. I imagine other people don't think of it much either."

"You're probably right," he replied. "But I just can't get rid of the feeling that I'm not normal somehow."

Roger knew that people weren't really staring at him all the time but it didn't seem to make any difference. He just couldn't lay the issue to rest. He had an unexplored emotional handicap much larger than the physical one. But he thought he had done everything he could do, that life was just tough and that there was nothing for it but to struggle on feeling depressed. And though the artificial arm he had was the latest technology and very functional, he never used it. He wore the heavy prosthesis almost like a symbol of the heaviness he felt, and kept the hand tucked in his pocket so it would be unobtrusive.

If Roger's pain really was based in an energetic memory resident in an immanent non-material field, then there was a good chance that a thorough exploration of the void might give him some new information, and even some relief. Roger agreed, and jumped into the work with enthusiasm, removing his artificial arm and letting us work right on the stump. I assumed we would soon uncover a lot of grief, not only because other therapists had suggested it was there but also because the cloud which hung over Roger was apparent to everyone. But it was not an easy subject to broach.

"Don't tell me I need to grieve," he warned me. "I've worked through all that shit and it's just not the issue any more." His antagonism was clear, and I knew he had distanced himself from therapists who had made such suggestions in the past, so I let the subject drop and hoped the void might give us the answer.

EXPLORING THE VOID

Within a few moments of entering the void, Roger started to laugh uncontrollably. At first, it seemed a startling reaction from someone supposed to be suffering from overwhelming grief. But gradually it began to make sense: through the accident and amputation Roger had somehow lost his capacity to enjoy himself. Life had become altogether too serious.

After one or two sessions, Roger felt a flow of warmth entering the arm, going down and extending into the phantom hand and fingers. A day or two later, the fingers of the absent hand, which had previously felt closed and crushed, began to open and stay open for several hours at a time, a feeling Roger had only experienced fleetingly while drifting off to sleep.

Over the next few days, Roger plunged into the void at every opportunity. The more he went there, the more he discovered the joy and aliveness he had suppressed or forgotten; and he often laughed ecstatically as he noticed new sensations in his missing hand. At the same time, as he got to know some of the other clients and understood that they too were injured and didn't judge him for being "disabled," he found he could risk coming out of himself. He rediscovered his playfulness and his love of story-telling; and he began to make whimsical remarks and play with words.

Roger welcomed the return of a part of himself he had almost forgotten, and soon realized that the absent arm had simply become a focus for a deeper malaise. He began to acknowledge to himself, that his loss of joy had actually *preceded* his injury, coming on over several years as a response to the pressures of a job, a mortgage, approaching middle age and a kind of creeping boredom. The injury was just the last straw, and became an excellent "reason" for the lack of fire and enthusiasm he felt. It just wasn't the whole story.

Roger's crushing phantom pain had become a metaphor for the fact that he was feeling crushed by life, just as the phantom hand's coldness reflected the coldness and isolation of his existence. His strategy was apparently to project all his negative feelings into his absent arm which, having been crushed anyway, could just as well contain deeper sorrows. Absolute denial of these wounds made it possible to go to work every day and exude the kind of confidence that he needed in order to do his job adequately. By localizing feelings in an arm that wasn't there, Roger could in a sense dissociate himself from them twice over and so doubly deny them. Eventually, the absent arm became the container for everything that was not working in his life.

RECURRENCE OF DEPRESSION

Roger returned home from his residence feeling like a different person. His phantom hand was much less painful and somewhat more open, as was his spirit. Within six months, however, he found himself sinking into his old habits of isolation and loneliness and, two years later, he returned to us, his recurring depression more of a problem than his pain. I was excited to see him again and asked how he was getting on.

"I'm okay, I guess, for an amputee," he quipped. I could see his dark sense of humour was still alive and well.

"How is your hand?" I asked, genuinely interested. "Is it still open?"

"You know I haven't really thought about that. But now that you mention it, I have to admit it's never clenched up again the way it was before I came here."

"You haven't thought about it? I queried, not sure why he had come back if his pain wasn't troubling him. "I trust that's good news ... isn't it?"

"Yes, sure it's good," he agreed, but as if on second thought he added, "But I'm not. I've been really down. They wanted to put me on antidepressants but I'm fed up with those guys and their pills. I told them they could forget the pills. ... I thought I'd like to give this place another shot. Sure ... the hand still hurts if I think about it but nothing like before, and I try not to think about it too much. But you know, its not totally crushed any more ... its partially open all the time ... and it has stabilized, thank goodness. ... Perhaps we can get it all the way open this time."

I remembered what a profound effect local xylocaine injections had had on Diana, the "sleeper" with the cat bites, and wondered what would happen if we infiltrated Roger's stump scar. Roger was keen for whatever we could offer, so we gave it a try. The effect was immediate: the stump warmed dramatically.

"It's working," he said, "my fingers are opening a bit more."

The scar site looked inflamed it was so hot, but it wasn't painful. In fact, Roger said it felt very good. At our next session, I ran acupuncture needles all along the edge of the scar site, with the result that Roger broke into peals of laughter.

"Oowoow aah!" he shouted. "That's the most amazing feeling I've had yet. Total electricity in my fingers, running right up my arm. I've never felt it like that before!"

"This is not hurting you too much?" I asked, wincing myself at the sight of a long needle running down the stump scar.

"I'll tell you when I've had enough," he reassured me. So we continued the stimulation for several days. By the time he was ready to go home, the limb was maintaining its new-found heat, his circulation had improved, and the fingers of the phantom hand felt alive and well. But more fascinating perhaps was the corresponding improvement in his depression which seemed to directly mirror the improvement in his arm.

## PAIN AS METAPHOR

The connections were not lost on Roger, who had one more question. "Everything we experience here seems to be interpreted metaphorically. Surely everything can't be just a metaphor," he seemed a little confused. "My crushed arm reflects my crushed life, its coldness reflects my isolation, its hiddenness my withdrawal." Then he let go the challenge that seemed to have been simmering in his mind for some time. "Isn't it possible that sometimes a cigar is just a cigar?"

Of course a cigar is always also "just a cigar," we agreed. But it is potentially something else, too. After all, an arm that is not there cannot just be "nothing" when it hurts but must also be "something." In healing, the metaphorical interpretation is useful in so far as it can help us to clarify our feelings. An injury very naturally attracts our unease and our fear. But it can also become loaded with other associated feelings until it is no longer merely a container of negative feelings but the active source of a negative interpretation of experience.

As we have seen throughout this book, physical pain can become a screen for emotional pain which is too difficult to grapple with. Pain related to an injury in time attracts our grief, our anger and then our blame. The more pain, the more angry we feel and the more we focus on the injured part and begin to blame it for everything that is wrong in our lives. Pain must be shut away, it seems. It seldom occurs to us to confront it. So, to examine the metaphors it contains — what it has been used to stand in for — can be exceptionally useful.

The experience of Roger and others with phantom pain may be more convincing testaments than anything else could be to the existence of an energy body, simply because physical explanations are not sustainable in the absence of a physical form. In my view, an immanent non-material field which stores experience, accumulates memories, generates thoughts and generally acts as a matrix for our inner life, provides a more complete explanation of the healing experiences we have witnessed.

I find it fascinating that since such fields extend beyond the body, then what we think of as "inner" is also "outer," meaning, among other things, that our inner experiences are probably not as personal as we might like to believe. Perhaps Roger's pain was a bigger metaphor than he thought. His pain was my pain and his grief and depression were also a part of me. By living as an amputee, I have a suspicion he somehow carried something for me — my fear of the same.

# Chapter 19

# POSSESSION

*Allow nature its mysteries because*
*mystery is truth's dancing partner;*
*because a respect for mystery may go*
*deeper than our knowledge ever can,*
*and because our knowledge, where it*
*pretends to replace mystery, may only*
*be an arrogant caricature of the truth.*

— Goethe

*A*lthough not acknowledged by modern Western medicine, other medical, shamanic and religious traditions have long recognized possession as a cause of disease. Scientific medicine has studiously distanced itself from such a notion, perhaps because it treads too close to religion for medicine's comfort. The issue is certainly fraught with fear. The idea that people could be taken over by spirits and lose control of their destiny is a particularly disturbing one. Urban myths and contemporary movies follow a long tradition by capitalizing on this paranoia. By attributing frightening and supernatural powers to these inhabiting spirits and by invoking sacred philosophical and religious concepts, they perhaps rush in where angels might fear to tread.

How do we know if someone is possessed? And what can we do about it? Surprisingly, my experience has led me to believe that possession may be quite a common thing and that it doesn't have to be frightening. In fact, understood in the context of energy medicine, the phenomenon may have practical applications, although a certain caution is advisable because outcomes may not always be acceptable. A personal experience and couple of case histories may illustrate the point.

## ACUTE BACK PAIN

One morning, while I was doing my rounds at the hospital, I went to see a patient in the psychiatric wing. I have never much enjoyed going over there and it is a bit out of my way. This particular morning, I was feeling rushed and irritable.

As I hurried through the hall, one of the patients I passed seemed to give me a particularly hostile stare. I felt vaguely uncomfortable but took little notice until three or four minutes later when I noticed a sharp pain in my back which, over the course of the day, became so excruciating I had difficulty moving about.

Since I had not done anything that might have wrenched my back, it occurred to me after a little retrospection that I might have "taken on" something from the man's stare; and that the reason perhaps I had taken it on was that we were both feeling angry. Apparently, I had somehow unconsciously "tuned in" to his hostile energy and he to mine.

That experience brought many things into focus simultaneously: the transfer of energies between individuals' electromagnetic fields; and how the connectedness of all beings might be reflected in the phenomenon of possession. I thought of all my patients who over the years had reported pains they couldn't remember acquiring; and wondered at how much I must have missed in the days when I saw the human body as a strictly delimited structural entity.

## GORDON : POLYMYOSITIS

Gordon was a forty-five-year-old black American who came to us with polymyositis, a rare auto-immune disease in which the body's muscles are slowly destroyed by the immune system. He was quite small with a light build and had especially long fingers with swollen, arthritic-looking finger joints.

Gordon had already explored many alternatives before he came to see us. He was unhappy at being dependent on prednisone and had systematically investigated all the ways he could of getting himself off it. He realized that the drug was simply masking his symptoms — but to stop taking it would require some courage.

He eventually came across a vitamin-herbal regimen which permitted him to discontinue the prednisone without going into a relapse. The regimen involved taking upwards of thirty capsules of herbs and vitamins every day and was terribly expensive but it was holding him. His CPK levels (an indicator of muscle deterioration) were stable and he was staying out of hospital.

Gordon came to our clinic prepared to explore his disease to its root, entering the void at every opportunity and learning to allow his own feelings to guide him as he went. What he found was almost beyond belief. Initially, he had seemed totally disconnected from his emotional body; then suddenly his first contact came — an upwelling of grief which seemed to emerge from nowhere and engulf him in paroxysms of shaking.

"What was that all about?" I asked him afterward.

He was slow to respond. "It was something that happened a long time ago." He paused for a moment as if he didn't really want to go on, then thought better of it and continued, "When I was about fourteen my dad committed suicide ... actually he hung himself ... and I walked in the room just as he was dying ... all blue ... there was nothing I could do. ..."

Not knowing what to say, I said nothing and waited.

"I watched him die," he added as his voice began to crack with another wave of emotion. "Oh boy ... I thought I had dealt with all that. I guess I'll have to think again."

Gordon didn't deny the impact of the experience on the child he used to be but thought that with the passage of time he had moved beyond it and got on with his life.

"I don't think anything ever goes away completely," I said as gently as possible. "Sometimes the body seems to harbour memories which the mind thinks are no longer an issue."

This certainly proved to be the case. As he went deeper into the void, a story began to unfold. In one session, Gordon's mouth began to fill up with so much sticky white phlegm that he had to exit the void to cough up huge quantities. Gradually, he figured out how to spit up the phlegm and return immediately to the void and eventually learned to stay completely in it while coughing and spluttering.

This phenomenon lasted several days and then cleared. In subsequent sessions, Gordon began to assume increasingly bizarre postures. His dark skin became pallid, his lips pulled back around his teeth, his arms reached out and his arthritic hands and fingers became claw-like.

That was when the light went on: "Gosh, you know what I think this is all about?" he announced shaking his head in disbelief. "I think I'm going through what my dad must have experienced when he died ... the sense of constriction in the throat, the difficulty breathing ... the feeling my head is about to explode, and the muscle tension in my body. ... I mean, what else could it be? ... and you know what? ... I have a feeling that perhaps the muscle disease I have is related to all of this somehow. It's like my whole body is bursting. ... It's like when I go into the void I become my dad and experience what he experienced."

I couldn't disagree. "Well, maybe there will be some change now for the better. If what you say is true, then perhaps your muscular problem will improve."

"I'm sure it will," he affirmed confidently; and then as if to explain things a bit more he added, "You know we were really close, the two of us, but I had no idea we were that close. We did everything together. He would take me with him on his field trips ... he was a game warden ... take me fishing in the summer, snowshoeing in the winter ... but he was never happy ... always melancholy ... could never really relax ... just like me. It's almost like he's still with me you know ... not that I believe in that sort of thing ...."

I wondered if his words weren't more true than he thought.

## JANET : TOTAL BODY PAIN AND FATIGUE

Janet was a fifty-five-year-old Russian immigrant who had fallen against a wall at work and hurt her chest. Though no one had been able to identify any structural damage, her health seemed to go steadily downhill: she became depressed, chronically fatigued, and complained of severe, incapacitating pain all over her body.

When she first came to us, she refused to let anybody touch her so we had to send her home after a week in much the same condition as she'd arrived, assuming we'd never see her again. However, two years later, Janet phoned and asked to come back, saying she was ready to work hard and participate.

One day when we were working together, I placed my hand on her upper chest near the site of her injury. Suddenly, she went very cold and started to shiver. Her face became contorted and she looked at me with the kind of snarling malevolence which turned my blood cold. Right away, I felt a strange tingling sensation in my hand and up the arm, and became acutely anxious. It was uncomfortable so I tried to shake it off but it only got worse. A moment later, my body was thrown backward a couple of feet, and when I landed I shook uncontrollably for several minutes on the ground. I felt a freezing cold wind, and later, others who were present in the room when it happened told me they had "seen" a dark shadow rise up out of Janet's chest and circle around the room before disappearing through a wall.

I was completely taken aback and lay in total exhaustion on the floor. The only remotely similar experience I have ever had was when I was electrocuted as a small boy, standing on a record player plug with wet feet.

It's quite possible that such experiences of direct energy transfer are the rule rather than the exception when we work with people energetically. No doubt most of the time the transfer is much less dramatic. Because the particular situation in question was so extreme, I was forced to sit up and take notice, and now am much more aware of the subtle influences of other people's energy fields on my own, and it is not insignificant.

In fact, since becoming aware of this external influence and its cumulative effect on my body, it's clear to me that I am constantly exposed to mild — and occasionally not so mild — forms of possession. The build-up makes for muscular aches and fatigue and if left untended for any length of time, can leave me very stiff. My sore shoulders, hips and back are intermittent reminders I must look after my own health or suffer the consequences.

Anyhow, whatever had occurred in that room, it seemed that Janet had released something and that something had profoundly influenced her character and behaviour. When it came out, it went through me like a cold wind and passed on.

After such an unusual experience, we did not really know what to expect but naturally hoped there might be some improvement in Janet's condition. After all, if Janet was possessed, then it would seem that de-possession — as it's called — might be a good thing.

But we had more to learn. At first, Janet plunged into a downward spiral and became virtually moribund. She complained of extreme fatigue and became completely apathetic for several days, hardly having enough energy to get out of bed. It was as if whatever had left her had been something so vital to her that without it she could barely go on. Wondering what would happen next, we observed Janet over the next few days as she literally "re-installed" her previous programming. Her energy gradually returned, and by the end of her time with us she was really no different from the day she came.

## POSSESSION AS A FIELD EFFECT

One way to grapple with an unusual experience is to try to describe and explain it in some acceptable way. Of course, an explanation does not change the fact of the experience but an intellectual grasp of something does foster a sense of safety and gives us something to hold onto while we strive to accept our experience rather than deny it out of fear.

"Possession" is just one explanation for otherwise inexplicable experiences. But instead of conjuring demons, we could just as well understand it as a manifestation of the way energy can move in, and between, living beings. An *e*-motion after all is just that: *energy* in *motion*. More than that, we often experience emotion in waves, as when we feel a "wave" of fear or of anger "wash over" us. And, like ocean or radio waves, emotion has vibratory frequencies, amplitudes and the ability to transmit information across a given field to where a "receiver" can tune in to it.

Possession may be no more than that, and an understanding of its mechanics can go a long way to explaining countless common and frustrating experiences. As we swim in an ocean of different vibrations and frequencies every day, we are so habituated to the interaction that we hardly notice it — until something big comes our way and throws us off balance.

The back pain I picked up in the hospital that day might have been a simple example of "tuning in." Gordon's experiences during our sessions convinced him that somehow he had absorbed some aspects of his dying father's spirit. And Janet's case woke me up to the consequences of energetic transfers in a unique way. But there was something about Janet's case which set it apart from other more mundane transpersonal phenomena. The more I thought about it, the more Janet's bizarre release seemed to indicate something of a different quality, as if the foreign energy involved was somehow self-conscious.

## CLASSIFYING LEVELS

Stephan Hoeller classifies possession by degree of severity: circumsessio (mild), obsessio (moderate) and possessio (extreme). "Circumsessio" represents those afflictions of the person coming from the outside which do not invade the personality; "obsessio" includes impingements on a being's consciousness and a partial interference with its free will and integrity; "possessio" involves displacement of the self by an alien, malign personality. The mild, or circumsessio, category might include otherwise inexplicable physical symptoms such as the back pain I acquired. It may also, I think, include common things like addictions and neuroses which afflict most of us to some degree.

In the moderate, or obsessio, category we may find deeper obsessions, such as being "possessed" by grief, or anger, or the past. There is much chronic illness, too, which I think falls into the moderate category. People who have been injured are often so obsessed with the trauma they feel has ruined their lives that they cannot move on. Such psychic immobility could well be understood as a form of possession. Indeed, persistent illness of any kind can become an obsession — chronic pain being a case in point — as the symptoms become a focal point of people's lives.

In this respect, Gordon's polymyositis had become an obsession, too, since he had thought of little else for some time. Only perhaps the physical illness wasn't the real issue — the underlying issue had long since been obscured by the passage of time. The physical disease seemed to be a pointer to something else, a metaphor for the deeper trauma he had tried to forget.

The third degree of possession — the one which sparks such fear and fascination — occurs when the energy absorbed is of sufficient intensity that it seems to maintain itself as a separate entity, sometimes capable of entirely overwhelming or altering the host, and blurring the bounds of self and non-self to the point of causing the host entity to speak or act like someone entirely different.

Until such energy can be discharged or removed, the host may remain unconsciously captive and behave completely out of character. Of course one has to be very careful here because distinguishing self from non-self is often a very difficult task. In some cases, the differentiation is probably a matter of point-of-view, even of semantics: it depends on what we mean by "self," and whether we are talking of "small-s self" or "big-S Self."

It would be singularly unhelpful to assume an energy is non-self when it may really be a denied portion of the self; as it would be equally unhelpful to assume an energy to be self when it is actually foreign. Unfortunately, there is no easy answer to this dilemma, other than to suggest that perhaps the contradiction need not be resolved.

## AMPLIFICATION OF DENIED FEELING

If we allow emotions to move through us as waves move across the ocean, their effects can be both exhilarating and cleansing. But denied or disowned feelings which are lodged in the body may well become amplified over time until we no longer recognize them as our own, and may well feel "possessed" by them. It is a small step from there to disowning them entirely and attributing them instead to malign influences.

Who should decide then whether we are possessed or not? Probably no one. Indeed, a conclusion need not be drawn if the situation is given the freedom to speak for itself. Perhaps the concept of possession should be taken as just one way of understanding an otherwise confusing picture — unfortunately an all-too-common picture.

## SELF-CONSCIOUS ENTITIES

Even the idea of a distinction between "energy" and "a self-conscious energy," or "entity" may be just a matter of degree. Janet certainly seemed to have experienced something of a different order than Gordon. Whereas Gordon was perhaps disturbed by a sense of his father's presence, Janet seemed to host a distinct, self-conscious entity in a bizarre symbiotic relationship which was mutually sustaining. The possessor provided the energy Janet needed for day-to-day activities and in return Janet provided a willing host for the aberrant energy. Thus, when the energy vortex left Janet's body, she crumbled and seemed unable to move at all. A few days later, she regained her composure and returned to her usual behaviour, leading us to speculate that the possessing entity may have returned.

## DE-POSSESSION

When a significant energetic pattern has been acquired, the pattern becomes self-sustaining, and remains in the body until it is consciously released in some experiential way. In certain cases, such as Janet's, there may be a distinct impression that the acquired energy is a self-conscious entity, but since that point can be impossible to decide, it is probably best not to get caught up in the dilemma. Often, a thorough exploration of the void will result in some insight, which will then allow us to draw our own conclusions.

Having said that, there are occasions when de-possession would seem appropriate and there are probably as many different ways of approaching it as there are healing relationships. Shamanic traditions often have specific approaches for removal of aberrant energies. We have tried a number of things — trance, hypnosis, matching the original vibration and shaking the wave form out. In acupuncture, the "Seven Dragons" — as the points are known — are indicated for this purpose. We now use those points fairly often in people with chronic pain, without making any assumptions as to whether or not possession is present, and the treatment will sometimes provoke a transformational shift.

Where the possessing energy seems to be self-conscious, then direct communication with the entity can be attempted. Obviously, a lot depends on the nature of the relationship between therapist and client, and some compromise needs to be found to get through the insoluble dilemma. Again, letting the situation speak for itself is usually the best approach.

TWO JOURNEYS

After his insight, Gordon felt confident that releasing his father's spirit would release his disease, so he attempted to do this with visualization. He was enthusiastic about the result and left us with high hopes that his polymyositis would improve. Unfortunately, that did not turn out to be the case. When we contacted him a year later, he was still having trouble, and had lost most of his enthusiasm for what he had learned with us.

Janet's experience seemed equally disappointing. Instead of feeling better after her extraordinary experience, she said she felt distinctly worse. Furthermore, after several days it was apparent that the possessing energy had reinstalled itself, and Janet gradually returned to her original condition.

Both experiences left me wondering at the complexities of the healing journey. I recalled a passage from the Bible which seemed to speak to the issue.

"When the Evil Spirit comes out of a man, it wanders through waterless places looking for rest, and when it fails to find any, it says, 'I will go back to my house where I came from.' When it arrives, it finds it clean and all in order. Then it goes and collects seven other spirits more evil than itself to keep it company, and they all go in and make themselves at home. The last state of that man is worse than the first."

We might conclude that in cases of possession we should leave well enough alone. But I doubt it. Certainly, a bit of caution is warranted, and clearly, we shouldn't be so naive as to think that de-possession is going to solve long-standing health problems. First of all, we need to be sure we are ready to relinquish our dependencies before we can give them up for good. Like giving up cigarettes or any other addiction, the temptation to return to old habits can sometimes be overwhelming, particularly if we do not have something more positive to put in its place. Indeed, filling the hole with something more positive is the basic principle behind Alcoholics Anonymous and many other successful addiction programs. In the case of "possessio," a similar approach may be even more important, while at the same time more difficult to apply, since people affected rarely realize the nature of the problem.

Just when we think we are onto something, life has a way of drawing our attention to how little we really know.

Chapter 20

# CHANNELLING

*In the void there can be talking*
*Without a talker, communication*
*Without a communicator*

The notion of channelling is another big stretch for the Western intellect. How are we to believe that our minds can be used to transmit information from "external" sources? The very idea smacks of medieval superstition. Worse, though channelling is in fact very different from possession in its effect and outcome, its process — apparent loss of control, contact with unseen entities — seems to raise the same issues as possession: the threat to our free will and the terror of psychosis.

It may be that the essential difference between the two is simply one of awareness. Some of the greatest musicians, Mozart among them, claim to have heard their compositions in their heads, as if the music were "given" them; likewise poets speak of being "dictated" poems by unseen "muses," and Edgar Casey's trances are well known to have produced extraordinary and accurate predictions.

Channelling has also been responsible for such exciting and enlightened contemporary texts as *Emmanuel* and *A Course in Miracles* — both supposedly containing entirely channelled material and fully coherent with the teachings of Jesus or Buddha. If these are the sorts of gifts which can be brought into the world by channelling, then surely it deserves a modicum of respect, even from the most sceptical.

I, for one, have learned by long experience and many wonderful and fruitful surprises not to look gift horses in their mouths: it serves no one's interests to discount anything simply because it seems irrational. Indeed, the many people with whom I have worked have taught me that total openness, without judgement, is essential to finding healing. Like anything else in this complex and awesome reality in which we live, the phenomenon of channelling appears to me to be something that just "is": neither good nor bad in and of itself but dependent on the understanding and intent of those who have the ability to channel — much as experiences in the void are.

## STEVEN : RECOVERY OF A CHILDHOOD GIFT

Steven was a 34-year-old man who had been rear-ended in a car accident and had subsequently developed chronic low back pain which had, over time, engulfed his whole back and radiated down both legs and arms. He had read a great deal about the problems of chronic pain and had explored a number of the various possible forms of treatment which address it. He had a good intellectual understanding of acupuncture, chiropractic manipulation and deep tissue work, and had been receiving regular spinal adjustments but nothing seemed to be helping.

Since his injury was not particularly severe, his unrelenting pain was hard to fathom. One would have thought that time alone should have healed him but for some reason he was stuck. By the time he came to see us a year and a half had elapsed since his accident and people were beginning to suspect he was malingering.

## THE SLIDE INTO CHAOS

Steven was a qualified carpenter, was married and had two children under the age of four. His accident had taken a terrible toll on his home life. In the eighteen months he'd been unable to recover, he'd lost his employment and was no longer able to provide for his young family. By the time we met, his self-esteem was shattered and his marriage had deteriorated to the point that his wife wanted a separation. In fact, she had made it clear she was only staying because she would feel guilty leaving him while he was in such bad shape.

Needless to say, Steven's position was precarious. His life was in chaos and he felt he had nowhere to turn. Though it was several days before he plucked up sufficient courage to really explore his symptoms with us, he was keen to do deep work. At first there was the familiar myoclonic shaking and emotional release but then came the first indication of something new; and, at a certain point, surprising things began to happen. During one session, Steven seemed to settle into a dreamy, peaceful state and subsequently described what sounded like an "out-of-body" experience.

"Where did you go when you had that dreamy look on your face?" I asked him after the session.

He looked directly into my eyes as if sizing me up to see if I was trustworthy and paused for a moment before answering, "I was hovering somewhere up there by the ceiling." He pointed to a spot where the wall met the ceiling — "looking down at what was going on. I could see my body and everything."

"You mean, you were outside your body?" I asked, realizing there was probably no answer to the question. But my intellect wanted to make some sense of what he was saying.

"Yes. I wasn't imagining it, I was really outside myself," he told me quite firmly.

I searched for something to say but could think of little. Eventually, I asked, "Weren't you at all frightened?" thinking that I would certainly have been. "You looked like you were having a really good time."

"No, I wasn't scared. You know it's not like it's the first time I've done it. ... I used to do it quite often when I was a kid," Steven let on, keeping his eye on me to gauge my reaction. "But it hasn't happened for a long time. ... It was nice really, took me right back to something I'd sort of forgotten about."

Its not unusual for people to go somewhere else during bodywork — their eyes roll back and begin to flicker back and forth as if they were dreaming — but few report being consciously outside their bodies. Steven's experience seemed to be qualitatively different.

Out-of-body experiences have been described by many people in differing circumstances — during surgery, near death, or during deep meditation. Near-death survivors have sometimes described an experience of "floating" somewhere above the place where they were severely injured, looking down at what is going on. These people often don't realize how they got out of their bodies but find the experience peaceful, not in the least frightening and strangely "ordinary." In some cases of serious illness or accident, people describe being offered the choice to either return to their bodies or move on and leave the body to perish, while others say they were told to go back to their bodies even though they would have preferred to continue their peaceful disembodiment.

However, Steven was neither near death nor traumatized; he was just breathing deeply, was completely in control and was enjoying it.

"Well, you seem to have a remarkable ability," I went on, intrigued but groping. "What's it like? — being outside, I mean."

Steven seemed to warm to my questions and began filling in some details. "I used to see these people — I called them my parents because at the time they felt more like my parents than my real parents — and I saw them again today. ... They were talking to me, comforting me really, telling me everything was going to be okay. ... They said that all this shit I've been going through the past eighteen months is okay. You know, it's the first positive thing I've heard in a long time."

He paused for a moment. "You see, they've always been around. ... That's why the experience today didn't surprise me. I used to talk to them all the time when I was young."

"Tell me, what happened to this gift? Did it just stop by itself or did you shut it down?"

"Well there came a time — I forget when — I guess I was in my early teens, I just felt it was stupid, you know ... thought I was making it all up ... and it just stopped."

"Did something happen to made you think it was stupid?"

"No, not really. It just became clear to me that what was happening was not normal — that it didn't happen to other people — at least, no one else I knew seemed to do it, and my friends teased people who were different. ... So I just decided I didn't want it any more and it stopped. Then after a while I couldn't do it even when I wanted to. ... So, in the end, I just forgot about it."

The recognition of his old gift turned out to be just the boost Steven needed and it was not lost on him that it had come about as a direct consequence of exploring his despair. He began to intuit a deeper significance to his difficulties and as he did so, something fundamental shifted in his psyche and his pain took a back seat to the rediscovery of his gift. And the more he welcomed it, the more messages he seemed to receive from his other-worldly connections. Gradually, Steven began to consider that the "shutting down" of the gift he had taken for granted as a child might be in some way related to his pain.

No doubt the exclusion of such awareness from his consciousness required a great deal of unconscious energy. And the resulting chronic muscular tension in Steven's body — evidenced by his cold hands and feet and unremitting anxiety — were wreaking havoc with his health. No amount of pain-killers, tranquillizers or other medication was strong enough to completely suppress his pain and he was slowly but surely being forced to a reckoning with this buried part of his unconscious.

Steven began to take advantage of the safety and support of the program environment to experiment with his rediscovered gift. One day, he took me aside and told me that his friends wanted to transmit a message to me personally. I was more than intrigued and we set aside some time. When we were ready, Steven took a few deep breaths and went into himself.

After a few moments his eyes rolled back, his voice changed its timbre, and for the next half hour Steven — or someone, or something — told me things about my life, my circumstances, my destiny and purpose which rung absolutely true though there were no specific details. In a sense, he confirmed what I knew intuitively about myself.

"Have you ever done this before?" I asked him after it was over.

"Yes, but not in the same way," he replied. "I used to get information from time to time but the few times I tried to pass it on, people told me not to be silly, so in the end I learned to keep it to myself. Actually, looking back, I think I probably scared them more than anything."

I felt truly humbled and privileged to be present at the re-emergence of this gifted man. He was exploring a new poten-tial and I was there to receive its first manifestation. We both realized the importance and impact of our exchange. Steven had overcome the fear of being ridiculed, had put a name — chan-nelling — to his talent, and so had taken the first step on a long journey toward health. Since he was still in too much pain to return to carpentry, he began to contemplate developing his new gift as a service to others. And as we both knew, in fact he had literally no choice if he wanted to recover his own health.

PAULETTE : OPENING TO OTHER ENERGIES

Paulette was a 27-year-old woman who had been injured when she fell off a ladder trying to climb up onto her roof. By the time she came to us, she had been in pain for some five years — mostly in her lower back and hips. On the surface, she seemed cheerful and well adjusted; the kind of person who saw the positive in everything. Indeed, she was almost too bubbly, always laughing and joking, and refusing to get depressed as so many people do when they have chronic pain.

"Most people don't really want to hear the truth when they ask how you are," she explained. "It's depressing to hear people moan all the time about their aches and pains. Much better to reply that all's well. Then there's no hassle, people don't ask a lot of questions and you don't find yourself pushing people away."

Paulette had chosen to face the world with a smile but in fact her smile was a mask. She talked glibly of "personal responsibility," and spoke enthusiastically of healing coming from within as if she already knew everything we could teach her. But despite her positive attitude, her back pain refused to let go and her pretence was wearing her out. It seemed possible that eventually she would have to acknowledge a deeper disharmony if she wanted to heal.

In the end, it took several days to get under her armouring. Early work with acupuncture had resulted in some myoclonic activity — a fine vibration emanating from the arms, legs and jaw. But then quite suddenly during one session, Paulette started reciting something which clearly had great meaning for her, bursting into tears every few lines and having to collect her thoughts before she could go on.

It turned out to be a poem she had written and, perhaps because it was her own creation, it somehow allowed her to pierce her mask and move deeper into her real anguish. The poem seemed to go on interminably, while Mary Joan and I sat listening and wondering where, if anywhere, it was leading. Meanwhile, her myoclonic jerking intensified and every minute or two became quite violent, as if she might be about to completely lose control. Each time, however, she would catch herself and calm down sufficiently to carry on.

But then something happened which moved the whole experience to another plane. Paulette's face altered in front of my eyes and I felt a wave of heat move up my back. The poetry continued but somehow took on a different quality. I wondered briefly whether she had just decided to let the words flow out spontaneously but moments later realized that it wasn't Paulette talking at all.

The voice had dropped and a clearly male personality was coming through.

The male personality looked directly at Mary Joan, sitting nearby and said, "This message is for you, Mary Joan, are you listening this time? I need to know you are listening." My ears pricked up as the situation intensified by the moment. "Yes, I'm listening," Mary Joan answered, suddenly curious as to what might be coming next. "I'm right here, please go on."

The male voice continued, "We were together for many years but when I left, I never had a chance to tell you how I felt, to tell you how sorry I was. I've carried this around for too long. I want you to hear me now so that I can heal."

"Who are you?" Mary Joan asked, astonished, but there was no answer. The question remained hanging in the air. After a few moments of silence, Mary Joan took the initiative.

"I hear you now," she said. "It's okay, you needn't carry this any longer."

"Thank you. Oh, thank you!" the male voice exclaimed, obviously relieved; and, then, as quickly as he had come, he was gone. All the time this was going on, Paulette was shaking vio-

lently but as soon as the thanks were done, her shaking sub-
sided, her face shifted again and she was back — somewhat
wobbly from her experience but clearly Paulette.

Later, she described the feeling of being in a cupboard while
people knocked on the door trying to get in. She had felt overwhelmed and frightened but claimed the feeling was not unfamiliar, having been a recurring experience in her childhood. At
the time, since no one had been able to put it in perspective for
her, she had deliberately shut out the messages.

## CHANNELLING AND FEAR

As channelling may elicit deep-rooted fears, it is not surprising
that gifted children find themselves and their talent rejected and
invalidated by adults and decide, consciously or unconsciously,
to shut their ability down. Why channelling should provoke
such fear speaks to the larger issue of "fear" itself, which tends to
arise when there is a threat to the integrity of the ego, even if
that threat is more perceived than real.

In fact, the ego is not annihilated during channelling, it just
goes into abeyance, so that contact can be made with larger
aspects of being. Perhaps what's really at stake, then, is the
destruction of the ego's illusion of separateness.

## CHANNELLING AND THE TRANSPERSONAL

During channelling we "tune in" to a transpersonal field. At this
level, we discover we are not merely personal but connect and
interact in a larger "field," in which individuals are nodal points.
Through exploring our void and consciously surrendering ego
control, we can learn to allow our small "self" to have direct
access to the larger "Self". Here, personal mind gains access to
information from cosmic mind. If we can let go and open up —
without fear — then the question as to whether the tuned-in
portion is "self" or "other" becomes irrelevant. It is only the ego

which worries about being invaded; and since fear tunes into and attracts fear, an ego's particular anxiety may well be a major factor in attracting less-than-welcome energies.

## TECHNIQUES OF ACCESS

To open oneself to other energies involves much the same preparation as to access the void. With sufficient practice and familiarity, techniques such as deep breathing and meditation create a fearless awareness and an open receptivity. When this stage is achieved, the body may shake or tremble, or there may be some other visible expression of an altered state of consciousness. The face may change its appearance or expression and the voice its timbre, while the ego seems to recede or drift free for a while; and information which it could have no way of knowing comes through.

The most fascinating case of channelling I heard about was a pair of cretinous twins who could, in the blink of an eye, perform the mathematical sums — such as multiplying two very large numbers — which would normally require a sophisticated calculator. It was as if they were just reading off the numbers, except that they could not read. Since they were cretinous, it might be posited that this unlikely pair of prodigies had very little intellectual resistance to transpersonal energies. Indeed, it may have been precisely their egolessness which saved them from needing to question and suppress their talents.

## PERSONAL CREATIVE POTENTIAL

Everyone has the potential to discover unique creative abilities through a process of ego surrender. As the stories in this book illustrate, such abilities can often be found by exploring the very pain or anxiety which for years we may have been fighting to ignore. Pain can be a doorway because it is a place the ego doesn't want to go.

STEVEN: EPILOGUE

For Steven, surrendering to his pain had certainly brought such awareness but he knew it was just the beginning of a long road to recovery. He realized he had to develop the gift he had rediscovered or risk falling back into chronic pain. And as if to force the issue, his wife did leave taking their children with her, leaving him agonized but free of distractions.

To everyone's delight, Steven showed up quite unexpectedly at the clinic about a year later. There was a warm glow about him which was impossible not to notice. He attributed much of his improvement to the study of Qi Gong, which had allowed him to move blocked energy and ease his back pain whenever it arose.

Equally exciting was his progress in channelling which he told me he now explored daily. His anxiety, his frustration, and the look of desperation were gone. In their place was a sense of quiet certainty and a willingness to share himself with others: Steven knew that he had found his path and an almost visible atmosphere of peace surrounded him. As he neared the end of his passage through the generative chaos, he had started a new relationship and was looking forward to the future with renewed enthusiasm and energy.

PAULETTE: EPILOGUE

Paulette, on the other hand, who had experienced a dramatic reduction in her pain after that single episode in the void, did not feel any particular urgency to explore her talent further and, for the time being, decided to simply enjoy her recovered health. As of this writing she remains pain free.

# Chapter 21

## THE WARRIOR

*Weapons cannot cleave him, nor fire*
*burn him; water cannot wet him,*
*nor wind dry him away.*

— Bhagavad-Gita

*M*oe was a 36-year-old communications expert for the Department of National Defence. His fifteen years in the army had been nothing but a success — top of the officer graduating class, regular promotions, top performer — he had never been passed up for a position. He seemed to be set to continue moving onward and upward.

But it had all come to an end one day two years before he came to see us, when Moe was sidelined by a car accident. In the accident, his car had been hit on the passenger side by a vehicle which ran a red light, and as a result he had developed an incapacitating neck and left shoulder pain. The pain radiated up to behind his left eye to produce constant mind-numbing headaches. As a result, he couldn't think clearly; he couldn't act in his usual efficient capacity, or do any of his previous work.

Over the two years since the accident, he had received every conceivable form of therapy — the military had spared no expense. But it was all to no avail. Moe remained in pain and became increasingly angry and bitter as he saw his promising career slip away. His anger did not go unnoticed by his physicians, who referred Moe for intensive psychotherapy. But time went on, and after eighteen months it really had made no difference — he was still angry, and he knew why, and no amount of talking could change it.

It was in this frame of mind that Moe came to the clinic. He was very straightforward, openly admitted his anger and scepticism, and pointed out that since he had tried a lot of therapy, we would "have to prove we were genuine" before he would give us serious consideration.

Cautious and methodical, Moe spent a couple of days checking us out before deciding it might be worth giving us a try. However, once the decision was made, there was no holding him back. Like a good soldier, he gave himself two hundred percent.

EXTREME SKIING

Within moments of his first encounter with the void he began to tremble, the trembling turned to shaking which progressed up his legs, through his torso, and eventually reached his head, which shook violently from side to side for several minutes. A short time later, he began to cry uncontrollably, as the energy released from his neck, moved down his left arm and out his hand. When he returned from the dramatic encounter, he announced the experience had been rather like extreme skiing.

"Do you mean like jumping off the edge of a cliff on a triple black diamond?" I asked jokingly.

"Almost," was his simple reply. "Certainly, a double black diamond — with powder snow!" he added with a grin.

Moe became intensely curious about his experience and wanted to go further. By chance, his acupuncture partner, John, had a similar disposition and affinity for skiing, and during the week there were many humorous references made to the analogy of extreme skiing. But that was not all. During one session, John lost control and punched the floor, sustaining a thumb injury I have only seen in skiers.

It was the first time I had seen anyone injured in the void. But beyond the injury itself was the extraordinary context in which it occurred. Never before had we talked about skiing and never before have I seen that specific injury except in a skier.

Moe continued his journey deeper into the void, each time shouting loudly, and shaking his legs, head and arms. His head shook from side to side, his whole body vibrated, and his hands punched the air as he exhaled expletives which would have done justice to any army mess hall. The swearing seemed to break through a wall in his psyche, and he began to stutter.

"Why do you th-think I'm fu-fu- st-stuttering?" he asked me.

I thought perhaps the energy surging through his body had met an adversary in his rational mind, which felt such language might be inappropriate.

"It seems something wants to emerge, and your mind is holding it down," I ventured without really understanding what I meant.

It was clear we had to keep going but Moe spoke of a wall of blackness and terror which he had not yet broached.

"I know exactly where I have to go with this," he said cautiously. "But I'm terrified. It's like a big black hole."

"Can you be very specific?" I asked him. "Describe exactly what the black hole feels like when you get close to it?"

"I get to this place where I start to choke — it's like I'm being suffocated and can't breathe. Then I get really angry. I mean really pissed — like bloodthirsty. I want to kill."

"Is this the same as the anger you feel from the accident?"

"I guess it could be," he acknowledged. "But this anger is beyond anything I can deal with rationally."

"Are you ready to explore it?" I asked, feeling a little terrified myself at the prospect of inviting killer energy to surface.

"Yes, I really want to get to the bottom of it. In fact I've already begun. Last night I phoned my mother and asked her whether anything happened when I was small to do with choking. She said the only thing she could think of was that when I was born the umbilical cord was wrapped around my neck twice."

While this served as a possible explanation for the moment, it seemed to me it did not really address the intensity of his rage.

## FOREIGN VOICES, OTHER REALITIES

"Before we begin," I said in all seriousness, "there is one thing you should know, which might help. When you hyperventilate as much as you will be doing, you'll have several minutes grace in which you can hold your breath before you need be at all concerned ... and it's highly doubtful you will go that long before taking another breath ... but if you do, just remember I can perform resuscitation if necessary."

That seemed reassurance enough for the military man, and Moe took a few deep breaths and plunged back into the void. Before long, he came to the place where he began to choke. I coached him through the choking, reassuring him as necessary, and he soon coughed up copious amounts of phlegm, breaking a block and opening a door which had never before opened. In the process, Moe never actually held his breath for more than a few seconds. The fear of choking to death fortunately never even came close to materializing. Instead, in the next moment something happened which catapulted both of us into brand new territory.

"Muefti!" Moe shouted, clasping his hands, as if holding a sword or staff, and waving it in a circular motion round his head.

"Muefti fuente, von schollenharten in fleckin tohorde," he screamed, bringing the imaginary sword down hard on the floor.

I was stunned. "Moe, you look like a samurai, or something. Are you speaking Japanese?"

"It's definitely not Japanese," he said speaking through his violent outbursts. "It's probably Celtic, German, or northern European. But boy, do I feel pissed."

He went back in the void and tried again. "Muefti von schollenharten...." His hands swung around his head as the sword crashed heavily down again and his head arched to the left, his tongue protruded, and his left hand went to his shoulder. He appeared to be trying to pull something off his shoulder.

"It feels like I have to get something off my shoulder," Moe said pointing to the place where he had had so much pain. He pulled his left arm frantically over his head while his head arched up to the left and reached an almost impossible position, without losing his ability to converse coherently. It was as if he could move in and out of the altered state at will — he could go in and experience something for a while, then retreat, gather his intellectual forces and regain his centre.

That night, Moe had a dream. He was standing in the kitchen of his parents' house, turned to notice the side door was open, and walked over to peer out into the street. There, in the distance, he caught sight of a motorcyclist revving his engine and looking at him. The rider and bike jumped toward him, taking off from a standstill in a perfect wheelie, skidding across the road and squealing his tires. As he came closer, the man appeared huge, larger than life, and was dressed in a modern day motor-cross outfit, complete with breastplate, studded plastic shoulder pads, shin protectors and boots. His helmet, however, was unusual: it was a full face mask, complete with a visor. At the last minute, just before he would have been run over, Moe watched the bike veer off to the left and smash through a large hedgerow, leaving a gaping hole. He woke up shaking in terror and sweating profusely.

Moe found great meaning in the dream, realizing that the man on the motorcycle represented a part of himself so terrifying he had never before wanted to acknowledge it. He also realized that now was the time, and he continued his forays into the void.

The next session, he returned to the moment where he was trying to rip something off his shoulder.

"I need to get something off my head. I can't breathe," he explained. "Now I see it. It's a visor or helmet of some kind with a pointed face cover. It's over my head, choking me. Either I'm trying to get it off or someone is trying to help me." While he pulled at it with his right hand, his left hand seemed to be stuck to his shoulder, immovable.

"Dueve taisn za fuego ter nuesen ore gianze!" he shouted, jabbing his right hand into thin air as if he was spearing someone in the guts. Moe then fell to the ground, landing on his left side; as he fell it looked as if he expected his left hand to reach out and break the fall, but there was no hand there to do the breaking. Instead it was bent up and firmly braced to the shoulder, as if it were either in a sling, or perhaps even cut off. He curled into a ball, and his right hand started patting his face with rapid movements as though consoling himself.

"Someone is helping me, telling me everything is okay. They are trying to get my helmet off. You know, there are several people here. One guy is like the motorcyclist. He's really angry. There's another bull-headed guy who's really stupid. If he saw a tree in front of him he would go right through it." He talked to me as if in explanation then re-entered the void.

"Kommen ya, kommen ya," he shouted, beckoning someone. Then his head twisted up to the right and he fell to the ground, grabbing his left shoulder. He lay on the ground writhing in pain, telling us he was being kicked repeatedly in the back.

"Ya fulfette stalton! Oh my God!" he exclaimed, as his head arched to the left. "They are trying to get my helmet off but they're breaking my neck. Why are they doing that?" he cried out. "Stoffen, stoffen dra dofen gieri. They're killing me! They're killing me! It's a mistake. They're trying to help and they've killed me."

Moe sobbed as he realized the implication of what he had experienced. Later, he related the scene to me in great detail. It was somewhere near the sea. There was a grassy bank scattered with rocks which sloped down to a shore where an azure sea stretched into the distance. In the foreground, right in front of him, was a small stunted tree with a gnarled and twisted trunk and a sparse covering of leaves.

Somewhere on the grassy slope was a large command tent of some kind, and at one point Moe felt he was inside talking to people. They were preparing for a battle and were reviewing the battle plans. He was pumped up and ready for action: neither angry or frightened but spoiling for a good fight. It seemed there were some tactical difficulties, and they were discussing what to do, as if perhaps their battle plan had run into trouble.

Moe looked wistful as he described his fighting instruments. "I had a beautiful sword. It was a flat grip sword, three or four feet long and three inches thick. My thumb could rest on the hilt like this," he said, showing me how he liked to hold it. "Solid … I really loved that sword, you know. I can still see it. I was the head dude, preparing my troops for a huge battle. But something seemed to go wrong. I don't know what. Maybe it will come to me."

"There was a second sword, a rapier really … also about three feet long …with a diamond-shaped hilt. … It came to a point and was razor sharp at the end. It was really light and I could carry it easily in my belt. And I had a huge five-foot-long broadsword … very heavy, which I needed two hands to use properly."

## SUSPENDING JUDGEMENT

Moe was a rational man. He had to suspend all judgement to accept his own experience in the void. Where did it happen? When did it happen? What happened? And what did it have to do with his neck pain? Was it even relevant to ask such questions?

I was aware of the trouble one could get into trying to explain void experiences. The most obvious explanation was that Moe had taken his own long military experience and expressed it emotionally with embellishments from Hollywood or his own imagination. The more mystical explanation, however, was that we were witnessing an ancient battle in which he had fought and died in a past life.

It was also just possible that Moe was channelling experiences not directly connected to him personally. There did appear to be a lack of coherence and focus in his adventures. He had seemed to be different people at different times: the motorcycle warrior, the brutish oaf and several others; and, in another incident, an Italian-speaking child, calling out "Papa, Papa!" To try to explain it all as one past life simply didn't wash, so we began to look more closely at the extraordinary language he was uttering.

I taped some of our sessions and took the tape to a linguistics professor at a nearby university. After close analysis, her best guess was that the speech was not ancient but rather a kind of generic northern European babble, with strong German and Italian elements that did not string together in any intelligible way.

As Moe was French-Canadian with grandparents from Alsace-Lorraine, it seemed reasonable that under enormous emotional pressure he might string together generalized northern European sounds — in much the same way a very young child exposed to three or four languages might, without making much meaning. Moe's bizarre language, then, would seem to speak more to his own origins than to channelling scenes from the past.

The experience left us with more questions than answers. I knew what I had witnessed; and Moe himself had no doubts about the altered but total reality he had visited. Once again, I realized that the world view to which these experiences point can be neither spoken nor proven; and at the end of the day, Moe himself could do little more than marvel.

What could not be gainsaid was the radical change in Moe's health. His experience had given him meaning in a way nothing else in his life had done. The more he explored the deeply emotional battle experiences in the void, the more his neck pain receded. In just a few days, it had grown nearly tolerable; and by the time he left us, he was a changed man, and he knew it. Gone was his blood-curdling rage; gone was his bitterness and pain; gone was his depression and hopeless view of the future. He felt ready to take his medical discharge and move on.

EPILOGUE

Over the next year Moe kept in touch with us, dropping in occasionally for a visit and keeping us abreast of developments. Although he continued to have some neck discomfort, his transformation remained solid, and his anger never recurred with its old intensity. After his discharge went through, he looked forward to starting his own business.

# Chapter 22

## WHITE LIGHT

*It ended …*
*With his body changed to light,*
*A star that burns forever in that sky*

— The Flight of Quetzalcoatl

*H*arley was an enormous man: six foot four and 295 pounds with a huge black beard flecked with white, and just the hint of a smile left, the rest worn away by constant and agonizing pain. He'd been a biker and a member of the Hell's Angels for many years and was no stranger to the tougher side of life but he'd hit the pavement some time ago. A couple of accidents and two operations had left him with little function in his legs and a very painful lower back. Harley was ready to change. He wanted to get rid of his pain more than anything in the world.

HARLEY'S FALL

At eight o'clock one morning during his second residential program at our centre, Harley fell. It was a little thing, really. He was getting up to go to an appointment and one of the legs of his chair gave way. He was, after all, a big man and the chair was old. He went down fairly heavily, landing on his sore back and within seconds was bellowing like a wounded bull elephant. The staff hovered around, monitoring the situation anxiously and hoping that his pain would settle naturally. But as time went on, his spasms seemed to become more severe, his bellowing became louder and other clients became uneasy. Eventually, the staff gave in to their anxiety and that of the clients and an ambulance was called.

When I arrived at 8:30, there were flashing lights, an ambulance, a fire truck and several very efficient-looking men in uniform. Harley was so large that the ambulance crew had felt they would need help to move him and so called in the fire department. They had followed traditional protocol to the letter, had started an intravenous line and were trying to manage Harley's pain.

Unfortunately, Harley size and circumstances were such that he had built up a considerable tolerance to pain killers over the years. The paramedics quickly exhausted their supplies — introducing more than forty milligrams of morphine combined with a huge dose of diazepam into the intravenous with absolutely no effect. Harley continued to bellow and his legs jumped and spasmed so much they tore the velcro straps off his stretcher.

No doubt the paramedics were familiar with the shaking associated with post-traumatic shock but it's unlikely they had ever seen such a display of myoclonus. Their training directed them to relieve discomfort by interrupting the spasms with drugs, but Harley was not a new client and we happened to have spent the past several days of his present residence specifically encouraging such myoclonic movement in him to help relieve his chronic pain. So he was not inclined to interfere with the energetic discharge he knew was beneficial. The attendants clearly had other ideas.

## HARLEY'S STORY

Harley had energy — lots of it — and he had been allowing that energy to move through him at every opportunity. But until this point, it had only moved significantly when he was in an altered state of consciousness, at which time he appeared to feel no pain at all. To allow movement while in normal rational consciousness was to experience his agonizing back pain while fully "in his body," so to speak. The present situation seemed to have forced a confrontation with an intolerable and overwhelming fear before Harley was quite able to face it. And, not incidentally, it had also forced everybody around him to face their own fears. How we reacted as a group to Harley's fall was to have a profound effect on the progress of that particular ten-day program.

When I had first begun working with Harley, about six months earlier, I could find no way into his emotional body using the usual techniques of acupuncture and bodywork. One problem seemed to relate to his sheer physical size, which made his body almost impenetrable. Gradually, however, we learned that his impenetrability was neither merely physical nor unschooled. Apparently, Harley had been so abused as a child that he had taught himself to shut out physical pain; and had subsequently put that tough training to use in his life with the Hell's Angels.

To date, Harley had been very disappointed with his progress. He could see things happening for other people and desperately wanted something for himself. I was equally anxious to see him break through but felt I was running out of ways to help. Finally, I decided to dispense with acupuncture altogether and try a bioenergetics technique instead. That proved to be a turning point.

The bioenergetic position we wanted to use requires the legs to be elevated to ninety degrees and held there until the body begins to shake. Normally, the individual holds the position himself but as Harley could hardly raise his legs at all, I slowly lifted them into position. At about thirty degrees, Harley let out a laugh like pistol shot and kicked his right leg abruptly downward, propelling me backwards into the wall. It was exactly as if he was kick-starting a motorcycle, using me as the kick-starter.

We tried the position again with the same result. As I dusted myself off and considered the situation, I wondered briefly about my safety and the likelihood that I would take on the pain I was helping Harley to resolve — a distinct possibility as I was supporting Harley's huge legs with my back. Something in me told me to keep at it, however, so I gently returned the legs to the thirty degree position again and pressed on, encouraging Harley to stay with it and breathe into the experience.

Several more kick-starts ensued, each accompanied by the mysterious pistol-shot laughter, until suddenly Harley's upper body began to shake, his legs started to quiver and his eyes rolled back. We called to him but he did not seem to hear and his pain seemed to evaporate into thin air. He was well into a generalized myoclonic seizure; and for the first time we could move his legs freely — even pushing them beyond ninety degrees, using traction — with no hint of resistance and no reaction. Harley was clearly in an altered or disassociated state. We decided to lay his legs down and wait, watching only that he didn't hurt himself.

He continued to shake for about twenty minutes and was inaccessible to ordinary conversation. He did not seem to hear us, or be aware of anything else going on in the room. Every now and again he would kick start with his leg or have a sudden convulsive movement, but for the most part he simply twitched and shook from his head to his toes. After twenty minutes, he took a deep breath and returned, as suddenly as he had gone.

When he was fully himself again, he was wide-eyed and awe-struck.

"I saw this light. It was so bright, I'd have to say you couldn't look at it ... yet somehow I could ... without any problem. Then I went down this tunnel toward the light and eventually I started ... I sort of went into it and became part of it. ... Can't describe it really. ... It's the best I can do. ... It was literally indescribable! And you know what? ... There was no pain ... for the first time in two years there was absolutely no pain. ... Only love and ... peace. I didn't want to come back ... it was so beautiful there."

There was nothing anyone could say. Harley was totally blown away, transformed. Here was the gentle boy whom life had so armoured he'd become unreachable. It was as though that flicker of a smile had grown to encompass Harley's whole being. I was immediately reminded of the tunnel and white light experiences of people who have been near death which I'd seen described in *Life After Life* by Robert Moody and I began to wonder whether Harley might have somehow had the same experience, even though he wasn't near death.

"I may look the same, but I'm not the same man I was an hour ago," he confirmed. "I've got lift-off!"

And change he did; he became as enthusiastic and excited as he had been depressed and morose, and his demeanour and focus altered completely. He was no longer concerned with the curse of his pain, but instead saw it as a doorway to a new and mysterious aspect of himself which was previously hidden and now promised excitement.

Over the next few days, Harley used the bioenergetics position to enter the light over and over again. Each time, he exhibited a variation of myoclonic activity; and each time, upon his return he attempted to describe the indescribable. One thing which was describable however, was that over the course of several sessions he began to notice a subtle but profound change in his body. His hands became noticeably hot and he could feel energy moving through his body in ways that he couldn't explain. More interesting still, he noticed that when he put his hot hands on other people, they felt the energy as healing.

Harley left the first program at that stage, hoping to return and continue his work at a future date. He seemed to understand that he had much more to do but felt that his next step was not yet clear. Anything seemed possible.

## COSMIC HOMEWORK

After Harley went home, two other falls provided him with opportunities which were to have profound consequences. First, his son fell, sustaining a potentially serious spiral fracture of his tibia; and shortly afterward, his wife fell, injuring her hip. In both cases, Harley had put his newly hot hands on the injuries.

The morning after Harley's informal hands-on treatment, his son's surgeon was quite astonished to observe that the boy's fracture lines had come together and sent him home without further treatment. Similarly, after Harley put his hands on his wife's hip, her bruises disappeared overnight and she was up and walking the next day as if nothing had happened.

Could it be that these were "healing hands"? And if so, what was the meaning of Harley's back pain and the light that he could "visit" at will? And what else might his disability contain? If the explorations so far had yielded this much, what else had we to learn? The possibilities seemed infinite, awesome and — for Harley — a little frightening.

It was at this point that Harley returned for a second program, this time bringing his wife with him. Eager and expectant, though afraid of what he might find, he was ready to go deeper into the unknown.

## THE EMERGENCE OF THE UNEXPECTED

The unknown came sooner than anyone could have expected. On his first morning back at the centre, Harley fell off his chair. To continue his story where we left off: Harley was eventually taken off to the local hospital in an ambulance accompanied by Mary Joan where he had a physical assessment and X-rays. Fortunately there was no sign of any newly broken bones, or other serious damage; he was just in a lot of pain from the trauma and associated muscle spasm. Mary Joan stayed with him over the next few hours, during which time he was given a total of two hundred milligrams of morphine and eighty milligrams of diazepam — doses which would normally be sufficient to sink a battleship. None of the drugs seemed to have any effect, however, and in the end it was Mary Joan's presence — reminding him to stay calm and focused, and to work with the pain rather than against it — which became the decisive factor when all the drugs had failed. Later, against the advice of the emergency physicians, who advised hospitalization and bed rest, Harley climbed into a wheel chair, wheeled himself to the door of the hospital, then stood up and walked calmly to his car, leaving the emergency room staff shaking their heads in astonishment, and at least one physician sufficiently intrigued to ask Mary Joan what she had done to help him.

Meanwhile, we faced a small crisis at the program, as clients began to react to the incident. We decided to suspend sessions and form a talking circle to clear the air.

TALKING CIRCLES

Talking circles originated with certain First Nations peoples whose practice is to gather in a circle to discuss matters of serious concern to their community. A "talking stick" is kept in the centre of the circle and the idea is simply that anyone holding the stick can speak freely without interruption or comment for as long as they like. When the speaker has finished, he or she replaces the stick in the centre of the circle where someone else can take it up. The process continues until the air is cleared and the issue is at least fully revealed and, at best, transformed. A talking circle allows people to speak from the heart without fear of censure, and in that sense it is very different from the sort of meeting most of us are familiar with where there is often a competitive, or adversarial element.

During this particular circle, two points emerged very early. Firstly, nearly everyone felt they should have been able to do something and were upset at feeling helpless during the crisis, even though there was really very little anyone could do, and all that could be done was in fact done very adequately by the paramedics. And secondly, there was a general feeling that someone should be blamed.

The feeling of helplessness was dominant and the defensive hostility we all felt at the exposure of our helplessness brought a lot of anger to the surface — which was then projected around the room onto whomever and whatever. It took some time before we reached the underlying fear — which we all shared — that despite the real suffering we had witnessed, all we could do was to be present with it and with Harley. We gradually realized that though we could be there and could empathize, we could not "fix." This process of exposure, although difficult, led over the next two hours to a genuine sharing of our common human experience of fear and helplessness.

When Harley returned later that day, strengthened by his experience, and clearly pleased at how he'd come through it by his own efforts, we were forced to reckon with the fact that the whole experience had been very good for him. That such an event might prove to be positive was something many people found quite difficult to assimilate, particularly as it was in direct contradiction to the opinions many had expressed during the talking circle. However, Harley's confident re-appearance — more than anything else could possibly have done — graphically demonstrated that those opinions had been premature.

## THE MOVEMENT OF QI

It is in confronting and experiencing our helplessness without looking for explanations or rationalizations that we surrender to the mystery of existence and can begin to heal. During the circle, at least half of the participants were visibly shaking. Exploring the truth of our feelings — difficult as they were — brought with it physical shaking — as "energy," or the Qi, began to move.

It is apparent that the Qi moves quite naturally, and without any effort, when we are willing to share our truth from a place of vulnerability. Like water flowing downhill, the body's energy flows in the direction of balancing as soon as we get out of the way and stop blocking it. An area of high electromagnetic charge will discharge to an area of lower charge, and in a group situation, this can translate to a number of people shaking or emoting. Although we did not realize it at the time, Harley's fall, by catapulting us all into our helplessness, initiated the beginnings of healing for the entire group. As the week moved on, we began to see the whole incident in its larger perspective: one in which the whole group's dynamic was involved. It was as if the whole thing had been engineered in some way by some unseen hand.

I suppose we will never know for sure but it did occur to me that if Harley really wanted to be a healer he had made an impressive start.

## NON-JUDGEMENT, NON-INTERFERENCE

Although his particular case sticks out in my mind, experiences like "Harley's fall" are not uncommon. Such experiences constantly remind me to reflect on the issues of judgement and interference in the healing process. The urge to fix, repair, or smooth over unpleasant experiences or conflicts seems to be so ingrained in our culture in general — and in medical practice in particular — that we find it very difficult to just allow things to be as they are.

We all have a bit of the rescuer in us. Yet when we intervene prematurely in other people's experiences when all that is really necessary is to be present, we can only make matters worse. This particular experience, however, really taught us something. We were forced to let the situation speak for itself and in so doing tapped into something deeper, something unimaginable at the outset. By being consciously present, without interference, we opened ourselves to the mysterious transformational forces inherent in every moment.

Of everyone concerned, Harley was the least upset by his experience: he was able to put it all into perspective fairly quickly. On the other hand, though it would be nice to say his back pain was better when he left us, it wasn't. However, while a superficial physical assessment might have found no significant changes, at a deeper level things were — as Harley himself insisted — very different: Harley's back was no longer his primary issue. His depression was gone and he had begun to regard his pain from a new and more fertile perspective. His pain had become a doorway to new worlds; it had become his ally.

"You know," he told me when we said goodbye, "my pain is really the same as it was. I can't say there has been any change, for better or worse. ... But I feel totally different inside. ... It's like I've put on a new set of inner clothes ... you just can't put this kind of experience into words. People who know me well will just have to look at me and they'll know. ... I can't wait to get home and see my old friends ... they are not going to believe the change."

Harley still rides motorcycles and has had more accidents since he left us. He seems to have a streak in him which likes high drama and risk, which from time to time gets him into trouble. But there's been no recurrence of depression or hopelessness; and, when appropriate, he uses the gift of healing which still seems to flow through his hands. It keeps him in touch with something larger than himself; it's a connection to the white light.

# Chapter 23

# MORE WHITE LIGHT

*Men often stumble over the truth*
*but most of them pick themselves up*
*and hurry off as if nothing had happened*

— Winston Churchill

White light experiences are happening with increasing frequency in the work that we do. Those who have them have difficulty describing their encounters, using terms like "indescribable" or "beyond words." Often, the white light is not something "seen" so much as it is experienced as an enveloping, all-embracing sensation of peace and acceptance. Repeatedly, people have told us that they feel this light is *not in any real sense separate from them.* They do not so much observe it, they tell us, as become a part of it.

Although certainly remarkable, white light experiences are nothing new. It is fascinating to me that our common English expression, "seeing the light," which refers to the minor "transformation" which comes with a new — and usually liberating — understanding of a situation or idea, may be a much watered-down version of this same profound and transformational white light experience, signalling humanity's long acquaintance with and acceptance of the phenomenon. Similarly, our word "enlightenment" suggests the sudden sense of "light" that comes with achieving freedom from false and limiting beliefs.

Harley's experiences turned out to be just the first of a number of clients' encounters with white light. But until a certain number had related their experiences to us, I assumed that we were dealing with another subjective experience, similar to other inner experiences — an aspect of the void encountered by those exploring their illnesses. Gradually, however, it became clear that a white light experience is something more profound than any other, that in fact it is really not an "experience" at all but a phenomenon so inclusive and complete that it lies beyond our normal categories — and so beyond accurate description — in a realm which cannot be imagined by the intellect.

To discuss this experience-that-lies-beyond-experience, then, is difficult. How can we speak about it? The intellect founders in the face of something beyond itself, something not just difficult to understand but something it *cannot* — and, by definition, *never will be able to* — understand.

### RICK : DEGENERATIVE DISK DISEASE AND A VISION

Rick was a middle-aged school custodian with chronic back pain from degenerative disk disease in his lumbar spine which was not amenable to surgery. Like so many other of our clients, he had been using antidepressants, tranquillizers and pain killers for quite some time and had ceased to imagine life without them.

Rick had strong features, prominent cheekbones, eyes which seemed to see through to some place beyond, and a great shock of grey hair. It was clear from looking at him that there was First Nations blood flowing in his veins and when we met, I was immediately drawn to his powerful presence.

He looked at me quizzically during our first meeting and when I asked him what he was thinking, he told me he was a bit taken aback to discover a physician propounding a philosophy he felt intuitively to be in harmony with his own beliefs.

### HORACE : ANGER AND PAIN

Horace was both fascinating and infuriating. He was a man who had delved deeply into eastern philosophy and had spent several years in India in an ashram. He had a penetrating intellect which he habitually used to expose the tiniest flaw or weakness in others. Unfortunately, he seemed to think everyone he encountered was an opponent worthy of attack and was quite impervious to the distress his behaviour often caused.

Horace radiated anger, and though it had distanced everyone he knew and put off even casual acquaintances, he did not seem to be aware of it. It was other people who had a problem. But for the development of high blood pressure and the sinister warning of a minor stroke, he would probably have remained oblivious. But the threat of further vascular events had convinced him he needed to take action to reduce his stress.

I could see that it was going to be difficult to encourage him to look honestly at his feelings instead of hiding in his intellect. Though it was very likely a factor in his vascular disease, he categorically denied his internalized anger, and so was quite unable to fathom his illness. Although he had spent years in India trying to discover truth and inner peace, the "peace" at least had not been forthcoming. He remained tormented; and as his health deteriorated, he worried increasingly about it without the least recognition of his own part in the situation.

## HEAD VERSUS HEART

As luck would have it, or perhaps as destiny dictated, Rick and Horace were "buddies" for acupuncture. Of course, who we choose to pair with whom is largely intuitive, and we can never know for sure what any particular mix of personalities will produce over the course of ten days. But recognizing two men on spirit quests — though their chosen paths seemed very different — we decided it might be appropriate to pair them.

It turned out to be an extraordinary combination. On the one hand, we had Rick — in touch with his own spiritual traditions and open to the inner man; on the other, Horace — a classic example of the mind/body split, a man who though well-versed in many spiritual traditions, lived entirely in his head and was locked into a world-view which, far from "saving" him, was actively damaging his health. Unbeknownst to us, we had the makings of a grand clash between the head and the heart.

During the first session, while we explained our procedures to the pair, Horace sat on a nearby couch looking interested but making it clear he had no intention of doing any experiential work which might get him into his body. He avidly questioned our intent, discussing the pros and cons of the procedure at great length. We answered all his questions patiently, realizing that to push him would lead nowhere, but as time went on I felt increasingly anxious. Rick was clearly getting impatient and I couldn't see a way around the impasse without upsetting one of them. Someone had to set some boundaries or we would have to split up the pair — and soon. I was actively reviewing the options in my mind when Rick addressed Horace directly.

"I don't care if you want to talk all day," he remarked, barely checking his irritation, "but you're doing it on my time and I want to get on with things."

Horace stopped in mid-sentence and, barely shifting on his couch, in a tone of total innocence, replied, "I'm so sorry, I had no intention of procrastinating — I just wanted to understand. Please carry on, I didn't mean to interfere."

With that, Rick lay down on the mat and began to breathe deeply, initiating a stream of events which was to astound me in the days to come. Within moments of the insertion of the acupuncture needles, he was laughing and crying simultaneously as his body began to shake and tremble. A moment later he cried out, "It's white — so white, I can't describe it! It's incredible, it's so light! There's nothing to worry about, Horace, you can do it. It's totally safe!"

We could add nothing more. Horace, who left to his own devices was too sceptical to believe that anything of significance might occur, was transfixed by the intensity and validity of

Rick's experience. He felt the extraordinary generosity of the near-stranger who a moment before had been struggling to check his impatience but who in throes of his altered state called to him, reassuring and comforting him in his own journey.

We couldn't have asked for a better pairing. Horace would have spotted a sham in a flash. But here was an experience which touched him somewhere he could not refute. Horace knew all about the "light" from his travels in India. During his stay in the ashram he had become thoroughly familiar with transcendental experiences — in others. He had heard others talk about it many times and was aware of the awesome power of the experience and the deep level from which it emerged. Though he had not achieved transcendence himself, he had been there many times when others had.

After Rick returned to normal consciousness, he told us he had merged with the white light not once but two or three times, teaching himself to come and go at will. Later that day, he sat cross-legged for the first time in many years. His pain, he said, was exactly the same as before but it no longer bothered him. He claimed to be a different man altogether from the person who entered the program a scant twelve hours earlier.

LEARNING TO LISTEN

Most of us have long ago stopped hearing the "inner voice" which can give us clues to our destiny. Chronic pain invites us to rediscover that inner wisdom, and for those who make the effort, illness can be a guide. When we posed this idea to Rick, it resonated and made sense to him almost immediately.

In a subsequent session, Rick suggested we meditate to find guidance; he felt sure he could access an appropriate altered state on his own. Little appeared to be happening at first but after several minutes, he had a vision in which he saw himself journeying over water in a canoe to an island somewhere in the wilderness of the West Coast, where he was to effect a reconciliation of some ancient inter-tribal hostility. As strange as the vision appeared to be, Rick knew exactly what it meant and knew that it was pointing the direction for his own future.

## VISION AND REALITY

As long as Rick could stay in touch with his vision, he could see that things were very simple but, inevitably, reality returned and called him to heel. Back in his daily life, he found the enormity of his task was such that it was difficult for him to not be completely overwhelmed by it. He had had an experience, he had been shown what to do and he knew what it meant. What more could someone ask who is looking for a way out of the throes of a chronic illness?

The path out seemed clear but when he stopped to think about it, it was terrifying. Abandon everything you know, says the soul, and live from inner wisdom — quite a task for someone who thought he had a little back pain which, if rehabilitated, would allow him to return to work. In fact, it was almost too much to grasp.

To the intellect, of course, such impractical visions and tasks are frankly insane. The cold light of reason throws doubt on the validity of altered state experiences and fear reaches out to throttle any attempt to live from the heart. An altered state experience may seem wonderful — cautions the intellect — but how will it pay a mortgage, or feed a family? The rational world is unforgiving and dangerous: keep your visions locked away and stay safe!

## THE AMETHYST

Just before leaving us, Rick gave me a gift, a small amethyst he had been carrying around for several days. When he gave it to me he said quite matter-of-factly that *the stone wanted to be with me*. He didn't say that he would like to give me an amethyst as a gift but that the stone wanted to be with me.

His choice of words seemed to imply that he understood the stone to have free will, like a human being. This attribution of consciousness to a stone rather startled me but when I held the small purple rock in my hands, I felt a definite vibration. I was both stunned and humbled and looking into Rick's eyes, I felt my tears welling. He seemed to be able to see right into my soul.

I took the amethyst home and somehow knew I should sleep with it under my pillow. That night, I had a very intense dream full of remarkably real, yet entirely unfamiliar, people and places. The dream was so intense that in the morning I remembered the events as if they had really happened. And each night from then on I had remarkably powerful, clear dreams — of disintegration and change, of beautiful landscapes, and of multitudes of strange people. My dream life had become as vivid as my waking life and left me with memories just as real.

When I took the stone out from under my pillow to see whether it really had anything to do with the dreams, sure enough, no vivid dreams. And when I put the stone back, more lucid dreams. It was hard to refute the evidence; and it all seemed to point in one direction. The amethyst was somehow opening a channel in my psyche which was expressing itself to me while I was in an altered state of consciousness.

It was difficult not to conclude that this beautiful stone was more than it appeared. It puzzled and even disturbed me a little that it had the power to so influence my dreams, and yet it resonated with something deep inside me. I was baffled and excited at the same time. No doubt something significant was happening — but just what defied my rational explanation.

What did strike me fairly forcefully was that the difficulty I was in seemed remarkably similar to our clients' struggles with the new experiences of bodywork. I had been presented with a new non-rational experience, something outside my previous knowledge. Should I reject it as an aberration, or accept the experience in its totality? If I accepted, I would have to admit that perhaps my assumptions about the nature of rocks needed amending. Could rocks be conscious? The question seemed too absurd to contemplate until it hit me that my assumptions were grounded in my own mind/body split. After all, if there is no split, then everything is a form of consciousness, and that which appears inert is just a part of mind that I do not yet understand.

For several weeks afterward, I explored this new phenomenon which had entered my life so unexpectedly and continued to have remarkable dreams every night. I discovered, however, that dreaming so intensely made me quite tired, as if I had not really slept at all. Eventually, I decided to balance the amount of sleep I needed against the uncertain benefit of a dream experience and discovered that by using the stone intermittently during the night, I could get both vivid dreams and enough sleep.

## RICK : EPILOGUE

Rick stayed in touch with us at the clinic. Over the next six months, he gradually discontinued all his medication and allowed his anxiety to flood through his body. He continued to have back pain but it no longer troubled him in the way it did before, as he generally regarded it as a messenger and teacher.

In the normal course of events, Rick might have returned to his job but now was forced to contemplate something much more vital. For the next little while, he struggled to balance his heart and mind, to find a way integrate his visions with the more mundane realities of his life. It was a difficult time, with many ups and downs. At certain times, he felt uplifted by his visions, at others, he pushed them aside and listened only to his rational mind. But he found he was unable to return to his old way of being without unfortunate consequences.

On one occasion, about two years later, he came to see me in some trepidation with a very stiff, painful neck which had manifested after he accepted a stressful teaching job, and had persisted for two months without showing any signs of letting up.

A little acupuncture helped considerably but in the process Rick shed further light on his experience.

"I know exactly why this has happened," he volunteered.

"You do?" I rejoined, intrigued to hear more.

"Yes," he replied. "I tried the usual route, you know, X-rays physiotherapy, traction, anti-inflammatories, orthopaedic referral, what-have-you ... and was getting nowhere ... and really it's all because I didn't want to look at the deeper issue, you know." Then he added, "The grandfathers have sent me a message to wake me up and get me back on the path. I can see them all sitting back and laughing at me!"

Rick's reference to the "grandfathers" signalled a conscious connection to his ancestral roots. He went on, "I've been overwhelmed with the sense of responsibility which seems to go with the things that I see ... and really, I just don't know how to put it all together."

"Perhaps you could reduce the demands of your visions to chewable chunks," I suggested. "You know, you don't really have to save the world, but rather ... by saving yourself you do the best thing possible for the world."

Then he laughed. "Yes, perhaps I have become a bit megalomaniacal." And with that, we both joined the grandfathers in their chortling.

HORACE : EPILOGUE

As for Horace, Rick's encounter with white light had left him in a quandary. He was aware of the power of the experience but he also knew it was not for him. Ironically, he was terrified that an encounter with such numinosity would endanger his heart and he didn't want to take the risk. Instead, he rediscovered the joys of painting, a long forgotten hobby from his youth, and began to engage the rest of the program participants in a playful discovery of intuitive art forms. He encouraged everyone to paint something on a single canvas, so that the result was a composite of everyone's input. The final picture was remarkable in that it showed a wholeness which couldn't have been foreseen.

We saw no reason to interfere with this unusual way of expressing himself and left him to discover his own path. It was extraordinary to watch him — after several days of pointing fingers and being generally obnoxious — begin to feel genuinely accepted and, as the days went by, become less and less angry and more and more spontaneous. Perhaps it was the first time he had ever been in a group which did not eventually reject him.

I don't suppose we will ever really know what factor or factors allowed Horace to become less hostile and more engaging. But that is part of the beauty and mystery of transformation. The complexity of a multifaceted holistic approach is such that it is not always possible to know what aspect of the program has touched a person's soul sufficiently to initiate the transformational process. Such uncertainty is the bane of conventional objective and scientific enquiry which wants to know the nature of the active ingredient.

But what if there is no active ingredient? What if every ingredient is just as important as every other? We are discovering more and more that no "whole" can be divided, that there is no specific active ingredient in any system and that the functioning of each part of a system can only be explained in relation to the whole.

Chapter 24

# THE ALTER EGO

*The meeting of two personalities*
*is like the contact of two chemical substances:*
*if there is any reaction, both are transformed*

— Carl Jung

*I* remember reading the story of Dr. Jekyll and Mr. Hyde when I was young and being fascinated by what I took to be the completely fictional proposition of one person housing two entirely separate and unlike personalities. Little did it occur to me that such a situation could actually happen.

Of course, occasionally people will behave in a way which seems totally out of character. Such unusual behaviour may well reflect aspects of the self which are deemed socially unacceptable, and so suppressed. Indeed, such energies — anger or fear for instance — often emerge during an exploration of the void, and seem to be part of everyone's inner landscape. But they don't usually constitute a whole personality structure, nor are they completely dissociated, as they were in the case of Jekyll and Hyde.

## DONNA : MPD AND CHILDHOOD SEXUAL ABUSE

Donna was a 35-year-old mother of four with a chronically painful right shoulder. She had worked at a checkout in a large grocery store and had pulled her shoulder on the job three years previously. Her symptoms were initially diagnosed as a "rotator cuff tendonitis" which was expected to heal quite naturally.

However, contrary to expectations and despite the fact that there were no structural findings on her x-ray, Donna went on to develop disabling chronic pain which prevented her from doing her job.

As time went by, Donna saw numerous doctors, went through two physical rehabilitation programs, and made two unsuccessful attempts to return to work, but her pain continued in spite of everything.

Why Donna was not recovering was a mystery but there were some clues, perhaps, in her tragic childhood. Brought up by grandparents until the age of five, she had returned to live with her mother and an unwelcoming stepfather, who resented her presence and abused her. Then, at fourteen, Donna suddenly lost both those parents in an automobile accident in which everyone, including a close friend, was killed, leaving her as the only survivor. Later, she lived with an emotionally distant aunt, and an uncle who sexually abused her for several years. She escaped that situation by marrying, only to find herself in yet another abusive situation. In one instance, her husband tried to strangle her, and threw her down the stairs, twisting her neck quite badly, and injuring her right shoulder — the same shoulder in which she now had chronic pain.

When Donna came to us she was in quite desperate straits. Soft-spoken and timid, she tried to be both ingratiating and unobtrusive in every situation. I first ran into her in the clinic kitchen where I found her cleaning up.

"Why are you cleaning up the kitchen?" I asked, wondering what kind of person would feel obliged to do that within minutes of arriving.

"I always clean up," she replied. "I can't sit still if there is something to be done."

"By all means feel free to help if you wish," I said. "But you know, you are here to rest and heal and you really don't have to do anything you don't want to." I didn't press the point further.

When it came to entering the void, Donna got started as soon as she could. She arrived enthusiastically at her first acupuncture session, listened to the instructions and got right down to work. The anxious energy I had witnessed was just the most superficial layer of a boiling cauldron. Donna was long overdue to give her emotions full vent and only needed permission and a safe environment.

During the very first session she started to scream.

"Get off me! Get away! Please don't hurt me! Why are you hurting me? Don't do that!" Her body began to shake uncontrollably as sobs and gasps of hurt and fear began to surface. As the process deepened, Donna acted as if she were trying to get away from someone, and several times crawled toward the corner of the room to hide under a blanket, sucking her thumb and whimpering as if she were terrified.

"You are safe here," I told her. "It's just a memory. It cannot hurt you now." We comforted her as best we could, assuring her she was safe, and encouraging her to keep that knowledge in her consciousness as she explored her inner feelings and experiences.

Over the next ten days, screams of rage and terror erupted out of Donna until I thought there couldn't possibly be any more, and still they came. Memories of strangling, memories of the horrendous car accident, memories of repeated rapes by her uncle, and much more, all came flooding up, wave upon wave, in a cacophony of terror. It was clear that the experiences that had left her with zero self-esteem.

During one session she admitted to an overwhelming "survivor guilt" which made her feel she had to apologize for being alive and needed constantly to atone for her sins. I wondered how could she blame herself for everything. So much of it had been done *to* her and all of it had happened before she was old enough to be in any way responsible. But I knew that children blame themselves for the bad things that happen to them and to their families. And although she was an innocent passenger in that doomed car and an orphaned child in her uncle's house, somehow she had decided that the accident and the rapes were both her fault. No wonder she felt she had to clean up every kitchen she came near.

"Why do you feel that everything is your fault?" I asked her one day.

"Because I'd often wished my parents dead," she admitted. "And then one day it happened ... my wish came true. My friend too. ... I feel bad about that as well. ... Why did she have to die? ... She was just visiting, and had planned to return home on the bus the previous day."

She paused for a moment before continuing, "I wanted her to stay another day so we could spend more time together, and I asked my parents if we could drive her part of the way home. ... So it was because of me that everyone was in the car." She began to sob. "That's why it was my fault. ... I engineered the whole thing — all of it. ... I don't understand why I was the only one who survived. I really don't deserve to live. ... Why didn't I die and not them?"

Such an overwhelming sense of guilt, coupled with an un-forgiving drive to keep busy left Donna in a position where only a disabling injury could allow her to stop and rest without feeling guilty. Her injury became an acceptable way out of an impossible situation, and the disability claim gave her security and a freedom she had never known before.

But perhaps there was another way. Perhaps now that Donna had an opportunity to explore her feelings more deeply, she might be able to find a more creative way out of the impasse. She certainly was willing to try, but the road to healing was clearly going to take time.

Donna returned home in a fragile state. There was little emotional support for her, either at home or in her community, and although some inner doors had been opened, she had lots more work to do.

## THE SECOND VISIT

When Donna returned six months later, she reported that she had continued to have disabling pain and had not been able to return to work. She had remained deeply depressed, and was taking large doses of antidepressants just to get through the day. She was however, clearly pleased to be back, and wasted no time telling me something she'd never dared to tell anyone else.

"I've no idea *how* to put this," she started ... "but I feel split down the middle, like I'm two people. ... I don't know how else to express it. You don't think I'm crazy do you?"

"Not at all," I replied, casting my mind back to another client who had told me something similar, and tossing out the story to her in the hopes it might be relevant.

But Donna's split feeling proved to be almost literal. She really was split — right in half — with a conciliatory rule-abiding persona, and a more fun-loving, risk-taking, get-into-trouble persona, just like Dr. Jekyll and Mr. Hyde. A couple of days later, Mary Joan and I were introduced to the alter ego, who had been hiding all along. On this occasion, Donna closed her eyes for a moment and after about thirty seconds a change came over her face and her voice dropped several tones.

"Who are you? Do I know you people?" Sarah's voice came across defiant and hard.

"What is your name?" asked Mary Joan.

"I am a tramp. You can call me Tramp," Sarah replied as if trying to shock us.

"You are not a tramp and I don't want to call you by that name," said Mary Joan, refusing to become one more abuser.

"Then you can't call me anything. I don't even want you to call me Sarah today," she said, giving her name away, as though unconsciously.

"So your name is Sarah, is it? Alright, let's just talk. I won't call you anything."

"Do you like my hair? Don't you think I'm pretty?" said Sarah, sweeping her hair back and pushing out her chest.

"Yes, you are very pretty, Sarah."

Then she changed her tack.

"Donna is a wimp. You wouldn't believe some of the things she's done to me. ... One time she put me in a closet for *hours*. ... You know, I like to have a good time. ... Donna doesn't know nothing about some of the things I do. ... If she knew she would just *die*."

According to Sarah, Donna had had several affairs during her first marriage. And since it was Sarah and not Donna who had those affairs, Donna would have claimed no knowledge of them. My mind boggled at the implications, and I began to wonder whether that could partly explain why her husband had been so brutal.

"I wanna be more in control," continued Sarah. "Donna won't let me come out when I want. So I get her sometimes, and there's nothing she can do about it.. ... Now, Frank ... he used to be in control, but he can't be no more. ... I am real strong now."

"Frank? ..." I interjected, surprised at the inference of another person.

Sarah spoke again. "Yes, Frank. He's hardly ever here any more. He used to be boss but now I want to be. He can't push me around any more. I'm gonna be the boss now."

"Can we please talk to Frank for a moment?" said Mary Joan.

Sarah closed her eyes for a moment, flicking her head quietly from side to side as if she were looking for someone. She didn't open her eyes, again, but her face changed, and her voice dropped still further.

"Frank?" I questioned.

"Yes." He/she nodded.

"What's your role with Sarah and Donna?" I asked, trying to figure out who all these people were.

Frank replied, "I came along many years ago, to try to bring Sarah and Donna together, but it's been a long and thankless task, and now I'm tired and fed up. They just won't get on with each other, and I don't believe there is anything I can do about it any more. I just want to leave."

"Perhaps we can help — I mean, encourage Donna and Sarah to take another look at things," I volunteered.

"By all means, go ahead. ... It's proven to be too much for me," he replied, and then he vanished.

Another moment slipped by and it was Sarah who was present when the eyes opened. We offered Sarah a bargain, suggesting to her that a cooperative effort was needed because Donna was so fragile she might become ill enough to end up in hospital, perhaps even on more drug therapy — which of course would mean Sarah would be there too.

"I *really* don't wanna be in the hospital. Please don't let that happen," whined Sarah. It seemed we'd hit a sore spot.

"We are trying to help that not happen but Donna does need your help. Right now when you take over, Donna doesn't remember what goes on, and then she does things which she can't explain, only it's really you that is doing those things. Maybe if you did a deal, to help Donna, you guys would get on better and she would let you be around more. After all, you have said you want to be softer and more like Donna, and Donna says she wants to be tougher, more like you. Would you, for example, be willing to take some of Donna's pain? It would be mightily impressive if her pain was lessened when she returned, and I'm sure she would be willing to make a similar gesture in return."

"I guess I could take a little pain, if it gets me what I want."

"Okay Sarah, if you are willing to see what you could do, that would be great ... thank you for being so helpful."

With that she was gone, and Donna shook her head a couple of times and was back with us. She looked shocked and frightened as if she wanted to jump up and run away.

"Where was I?" asked Donna.

"We were just talking to a couple of people you know, and who were here — Frank and Sarah. Sarah suggested she might be willing to help with your pain, if you would be willing to let her be a bit more present. How is your shoulder, by the way?"

"It feels warm, and my head isn't so bad. Incredible!"

Perhaps Sarah had helped already.

Donna arrived at her next acupuncture session quite excited. Now that she had talked about her other half, for the first time she felt she might be able to heal the split which had plagued her for so long. She took some deep breaths, and fairly quickly entered the void, contacting Sarah at a barrier she had never been able to cross.

"I can see Sarah. She is bending over looking away from me but she's out of reach ... I can't reach her ... I wish I could just touch her."

Then her eyes flickered back and forth as an internal shift took place, and moment later we heard exactly the same longing from Sarah.

"I saw Donna just now and tried to touch her but I couldn't reach. It's a pain not being able to get close to her."

Just for an instant I personally felt the pain of their separation. It was right there, hanging in the air, just like the physical pain in their shoulder. Perhaps the pain itself was just a metaphor for the experience of *reaching out and never touching any-*

*thing*. After all, to be separated from the self is the ultimate pain, the pain we all have, but refuse to acknowledge, face, or feel.

It seemed an appropriate time to approach Frank again and talk of rapprochement but it turned out he was no longer there.

Sarah explained, "Frank's not here any more. He's gone." And then surprisingly, she added, "Hang on — he left a message." There was a short pause. "Frank says since he's no longer needed, he has gone on to help someone else."

Okay, I thought, so Frank left a note. ... I wondered half jokingly if it was on the fridge or the hall table. The whole situation was so bizarre, why not a fridge or hall table too? ... and anyway, who or what was Frank? He seemed to be quite different from Sarah and Donna, who were clearly related to each other. But there was no easy answer to the question.

## MULTIPLE OR NOT?

How does one react to this kind of experience? One could label it as a form of "multiple personality" but the label wouldn't do justice to the texture of Donna/Sarah's experience which seen in the context of their life, made a strange kind of sense.

We worked with Donna intermittently over the next six months, as and when she was able to visit us. A slow integration took place, with Donna becoming increasingly conscious of her alter ego. One major hurdle was allowing consciousness of some of Sarah's sexual exploits. Donna had considered herself morally pristine — a woman who would never have affairs or cheat on her husband. Yet the reality was she had had several liaisons — or at least Sarah had, but of course at some level they were both the same person.

"I felt Sarah coming into my body," said Donna one morning. "And now she is with me all the time. I can feel her energy inside me, inside me and a part of me. ... Now I feel like a whole person."

It was the turning point. Increasingly thereafter, Donna and Sarah appeared together. Donna began to express more of Sarah's characteristics, and began to lose the reticent persona she had initially presented with. By this time Donna's shoulder pain, though still present, was hardly the issue. Much more compelling ideas had entered her awareness. Indeed, over time, her pain became an insignificant part of the totality of her integrated self.

## DONNA: EPILOGUE

As Donna's pain gradually receded, she knew she was going to have to face the issue of her continuing disability payments, something she was loath to do because of the convenience, and because as long as she remained in pain, her financial security was assured. She put things off as long as possible, until pressures mounted from the insurance company and she decided she would return to school and complete her high school education.

After that we didn't see Donna for quite some time. Then one day about two years later she dropped into the clinic unannounced, and brought us up to date. She told us she had finished her grade twelve as planned, and was now working part-time in a secretarial position. She was in a new relationship which was working well, and her shoulder pain, though still present if she thought about it, was no longer interfering with her life.

Perhaps more importantly, she told us that she no longer felt split down the middle.

# Chapter 25

## MULTIPLE PERSONALITIES

*There is no such thing as a person ... only restrictions and limitations. As long as we imagine ourselves to be separate personalities, one quite apart from another, we cannot grasp reality, which is essentially impersonal.*

— Sri Nisargadatta Maharaj

*M*ultiple personality disorder (MPD) — before it was reclassified as a dissociative disorder — was described in the medical literature as: "the ongoing co-existence of relatively consistent but alternating separate identities, plus recurrent episodes of memory distortion, frank amnesia, or both." According to the textbooks, in MPD there is usually a primary personality which handles most day-to-day situations, and then there are secondary personalities which emerge in specific circumstances. The primary personality may have no memory of the times when alternate personalities are in control, experiencing the episodes as a discontinuity, a "blanking out," or at the very least, a time lapse.

The whole idea of MPD stretches credulity. However, working with Mary Joan — who has great insight in this area — has helped me realize that multiples may be much more common than we think, and that chronic pain — as we have seen in Donna's case — may be a signal of the syndrome. Sufferers like Donna, for obvious reasons, have normally been careful to obscure their real plight and are often so successful that physicians and even psychiatrists often practice for a lifetime without knowingly encountering a single case.

I might have counted myself among those people, the sceptic in me repeatedly turning a blind eye to phenomena which challenged my worldview. But over the past several years I have grown increasingly open to the unusual, to the point that people will occasionally risk telling me about their divided selves. I now realize that the existence of multiple personalities can only be a matter of debate to those who haven't encountered it.

## CATHY : JULIE, GRIST AND JOAN

Donna's one or two personalities seemed modest and manageable in retrospect when we met Cathy. Cathy was a 35-year-old mother of two who had been injured in a car accident several years before. By the time she came to us, she had been wearing a cervical collar for eighteen months, was habituated to large doses of antidepressants, pain killers and muscle relaxants, and was using a TENS (trans-cutaneous electrical neuro-stimulator) machine on her back almost constantly. Though her condition seemed to have plateaued, remaining essentially unchanged for some time, no one had suggested that she might successfully decrease her medications and recover some physical function.

When Cathy first walked through the door, I was impressed by the more than usual stiffness in her neck, which was completely rigid. Since there were other people in the car who were completely unhurt, I wondered why Cathy had been so badly affected.

"There's certainly more than meets the eye to your neck pain," I remarked, feeling very curious. "I don't think I've ever seen a neck quite so stiff."

"What do you mean by that?" said Cathy defensively. "I hope you're not going to tell me it's all in my head, like the others."

I realized I had better back off a bit.

"I didn't mean that at all," I said. "What I meant was that I'd assume that it's going to take a lot of work for you to get better."

I could feel Cathy was not convinced and wondered when she left if that would be the last we would see of her. So when she showed up a few months later I was quite surprised. From what she told me, my impulsive remark had really put her off but desperation had forced her to overcome her irritation.

Cathy fervently wanted to get well but was now clearly very nervous of me, and very reluctant to try acupuncture. Her situation, however, left her little choice and as we immediately recognized, there was no reluctance in her body. The insertion of the first needle brought marked myoclonic shaking which the nervous Cathy found quite terrifying. We did our best to reassure her and — as though the reassurance had been effective — the trembling settled down quite quickly and she seemed to feel fine.

The next morning when our paths crossed, I took the opportunity to be as friendly and as cheerful as possible.

"Good morning," I said, smiling at her.

She just glared at me. "You can fuck right off!" she shot back. "What's so good about it?!" The vehemence was explosive.

I beat a hasty retreat, wondering what I could have done to so offend her, at the same time reflecting that it was probably nothing to do with me and that, as I had suspected, there was a lot more to the woman than met the eye. It never occurred to me, however, that I wasn't talking to Cathy at all.

Later on that day, Cathy seemed to have returned to her usual self so I felt it was safe to broach the subject of the morning.

"What was going on this morning?" I asked innocently. "Did something upset you?"

"I don't remember anything" she replied. "Why, what did I do? I hope I wasn't rude, was I?" She sounded apologetic.

"You don't recall meeting me in the hall this morning?" I said, somewhat astonished.

"No, I don't," she replied.

"But it was only a couple of hours ago."

"I'm sorry," she said. "Ever since the accident I've had trouble remembering things. It's really embarrassing."

Not sure what to say next, I recounted roughly what had transpired that morning, sparing her the exact phrasing.

Cathy was mortified at her rudeness but could offer no explanation. Later she admitted to frequent episodes of "blanking out," in which she could not remember anything for hours at a time nor account for her behaviour.

"Sometimes I find myself somewhere, like downtown, without knowing how I got there," she told me one day.

"How can that be?" I asked her.

"I have no idea," she replied. "But it happens."

Cathy's husband, Frank, confirmed there were times she behaved totally out of character, as if she were another person. Sometimes, he said she wouldn't even recognize him, and several times she had been quite violent.

"How would you like to explore some of these blanking out episodes, and see if you can learn anything about them," I suggested. "You know, sometimes it is possible to retrieve lost information through bodywork."

"I'm not sure I'm ready," she said. "It's too terrifying."

"Well, whenever you feel ready let us know and we'll do what we can." I wanted to emphasize that she could decide when and how to start the work of healing.

A few days later Frank phoned to say that Cathy had had one of her "spells," and had become alarmingly violent. Wielding a knife, she had backed Frank into a corner and threatened mayhem. He had just managed to get to a phone to call for help. Both the police and her doctor had arrived, and by the time I got there, plans were being made to put Cathy into the local psychiatric hospital until she settled down. Cathy, however, had other plans.

"Get away from me, you buggers! Leave me alone. Let me talk to Mary Joan, or I'll fucking kill the lot of you," she announced. Since she was still carrying the knife, it seemed like a good idea. Moreover, Cathy clearly trusted Mary Joan and their relationship had to be nurtured.

When Mary Joan arrived she faced a quandary. It was clear that Cathy was asking for something beyond psychiatry, beyond medicine, beyond simple suppression of her symptoms. On the other hand, there were a number of people present who were prepared to force Cathy into custody in order to get control of a difficult situation. But that kind of control meant an all-too-familiar betrayal to Cathy — she made that perfectly clear. She was staking a claim for the right to heal, the right to be heard, the right to tell her story, and a decision had to be made right there.

"Keep those people away from me," Cathy said to Mary Joan.

"Okay," said Mary Joan. "But I need to be able to trust you. Put the knife down and I promise you won't go to hospital." With that promise, Mary Joan elected to take on a terrific responsibility but it seemed the right thing to do at the time.

Then looking at everyone present she added, "Leave her with me. ... I will look after the situation."

There was an attentive pause as the energy in the room changed. Within a few minutes the situation was de-fused and Cathy calmed down. Her doctor was impressed enough that he relented on his plan of hospital admission and decided to see what would develop.

Cathy continued to work with us. As her trust gradually increased, she felt ready to allow us to be present as she explored her episodes of "blanking out." During the first few sessions, nothing seemed out of the ordinary. She exhibited the customary myoclonic shaking associated with energy discharge and emotional release. With some practice, she began to feel safe with the process and became adept at bringing herself to the entrance to the void, at which point she felt something signal the entry into deeper levels of experience — and the onset of terror. There she had to choose, every time, whether to back off and stay safe, or to go forward and risk annihilation and loss of memory on recovering herself — if indeed she ever did recover herself. It took considerable bravery for her to persist.

But she was determined. During one particular session, there was a palpable shift in the room, and Cathy's face changed suddenly and dramatically. Her mouth became contorted and belligerent, and she began to swear. She looked and sounded like a completely different person.

In the presence of totally new experience, with no reference points for guidance, particularly when something significant and profound is going on, there is usually nothing to do except watch and wait, to see what will happen next. We have learned to have total trust in the healing journey. In fact, the terror of the unknown is often strangely allied with an inner certainty that everything is just as it should be.

"I have to get out of here," Cathy said. "Let me go!"

"Hang on a minute," I coaxed, rather lamely, not knowing what else to say. But Mary Joan was right there, holding Cathy tightly and keeping her present in the room.

"You are totally safe," she said. "We're not going to harm you, Cathy. Tell us what's going on." But Cathy could not be placated.

"You can both fuck off," she told us indignantly. "I don't have to stay here if I don't want. You can't make me. I'll do what I want."

"Cathy, you are quite safe here. You don't have to go anywhere. Please stay here and talk to us," I tried again.

"Why should I?" she asked defiantly. "And anyway my name is not Cathy."

"Well, what is your name then?" asked Mary Joan.

"Why the hell should I tell you?" she retorted.

"I like to know who I'm talking to," replied Mary Joan very gently. "And anyway, if I am to trust you, I want to know."

"Well, if you really must know, I'm Julie," she admitted.

A shiver went up my spine as I realized what was happening. "Julie" — whoever she was — probably did not divulge her identity to just anyone. She must have felt safe enough to tell us.

That was the start of a huge unravelling. A short time after Julie's appearance, other secondary personalities began to appear. One by one, over a period of several weeks, a whole series of personalities emerged as we visited areas of Cathy's experience previously hidden from everyone. Julie, it seemed, was an angry and defensive person who was Cathy's protector. She was usually very rude and obnoxious, telling everyone off in the coarsest language, and making sure people kept their distance. When Julie showed up, Cathy completely disappeared, and when Cathy returned, she had no memory of what had occurred.

Another persona was Joan, a terrified little girl of about five, who spent her time hiding in a cupboard.

"It's dark in here," she would cry repeatedly. "How come I gotta stay here? I'm bad. Mum says I'm bad. She's gonna find me."

"You are not bad, and you don't have to stay in there. Why don't you come out?"

"I *can't!*" she emphasized. "Mum would kill me, and anyway, Grist won't let me."

Grist was another sub-personality, a caretaker who looked after all the different personalities and made sure everything hung together without Cathy's knowledge. We contacted Grist on another occasion. She was a more organized type, and was quite used to juggling everything around to keep the peace. She was definitely feeling the pinch.

"Why don't you let Cathy in on all of this instead of taking it all on yourself?" I asked her one day.

"Cathy doesn't want to know," said Grist. "She's a wimp, she always leaves me to handle everything difficult. She really pisses me off. Whenever the going gets tough, she takes off. She's forever pretending not to know anything about us."

"Why do you make Joan stay in the cupboard?" I asked.

"I don't," she told us. "Joan just seems to like it in there. I've suggested she come out but she won't. She's too frightened of her mother, and there's really no reasoning with her. I've tried."

"But her mother's not around any more," I countered.

"True," said Grist, without taking the idea any further.

Such bizarre conversations became quite commonplace. The sub-personalities volunteered different names, abilities, behaviours, attitudes, ways of speaking, and symptoms. Joan was a little girl; several others were angry and abusive; Grist, a caretaker. Some personalities were physically injured, like Cathy, and some weren't. (It is fascinating to me as a practitioner that sometimes the different personalities manifest totally different illnesses. For example, it is not uncommon for one to have diabetes; a second, food allergies; a third, back pain; and so on. Donna, we recall, had shoulder pain while Sarah did not.)

There were as many as ten personas in all and as time went on we had to befriend each one separately. Just when we thought we had gained a little trust, another personality would appear who claimed not to know us, and often didn't want to. Eventually, we felt as though we were running a kind of committee meeting, encouraging the various personalities to communicate.

## HOW DOES IT HAPPEN?

Some children, tragically, grow up in situations so bizarre as to provoke disbelief in those who hear their stories. It's generally believed that when children grow up in an environment where abuse is severe, or prolonged, or where the child feels there is no possibility of help or understanding from outside (as is often the case with ritual abuse sufferers) the development of multiple personalities provides the only possible escape.

In Cathy's case, her biological father had left when she was very young and she was brought up by an emotionally unstable mother and a string of stepfathers, some of whom physically and sexually abused her. For children like her, there seems no recourse, no place of safety. Should they ask for help, they are usually not believed, and find themselves repeatedly betrayed by adults. To them, the world is so hostile they have no option but to retreat into themselves and develop strategies to dissociate from experiences too terrifying to allow into their consciousness. By creating entirely separate personalities with whom they have no conscious association, they can learn to confront and participate in intolerable situations then "blank them out," saving their primary personality from having to face them.

In *Ritual Abuse, What It Is and Why It Happens,* Margaret Smith discusses multiple personalities in disturbed children. One common personality she describes is the "internalized perpetrator," a self-flagellating personality who identifies with the real-life abuser. By adopting the abuser's point of view, the child can dissociate from her own emotions, and endure maltreatment. That same internalized perpetrator, however, may become the blueprint for the next generation's adult abuser.

Another one is the "protector," a character who functions to keep the child safe at any cost, without regard for others. Like Cathy's Julie, the protector is the child's advocate, who sets up defences which effectively keep everyone at arm's length. Most multiples have a dominant personality who is presentable and can function in the day-to-day world and keep other personalities under wraps. These characters are often completely amnesic about any negative childhood experiences.

Then there are "intellectual" personalities who are aware of the childhood experience but who are emotionally detached from it and adept at avoiding its pain. More sinister still are the seriously deviant characters, the "killer," the "torturer," and the "rapist," who arise in extreme circumstances and may be entirely without remorse. These personalities develop to act

out the rage which the primary personality has not only repressed but with which it is entirely out of touch.

The emergence of these violent personalities in therapy can
be terrifying for both client and therapist. When confronted with
a killer persona, therapists find themselves caught in an ethical
dilemma of considerable magnitude: they have little choice but to
report the client, all the while knowing that this repeats the original betrayal and will block all possible future integration.

Balancing the deviant negative personalities are the sweet,
angelic personas. As society is more accepting of these characters, they tend to become dominant, relegating the negatives to a
subordinate, subconscious position much of the time. These
"nice" personas may have little awareness of the monsters lurk-
ing in their depths. When they are aware, the shame they feel
may lead them to project the evil onto others. The more complete the dissociation, the more the "sweetness and light" persona may be incapable of identifying the evil which lies within.

## A HOLISTIC MODEL

I believe a multi-dimensional, or holistic, model of the multiple
personality can shed light on this fascinating syndrome. If we
consider that each manifested personality represents a *unique
multi-dimensional solution to the problem of an individual's existence,* as one possibility amongst others, we can see that each is, to
all intents and purposes, a different person. Perhaps that is why it
is so difficult for multiples to integrate and heal.

For Cathy, entering the void repeatedly did not immediately
lead to integration. First came an increasing consciousness of
long-lost parts of herself, then a period during which she began
to piece together a relationship between her "selves," then a long
period during which she slowly learned to recall the gaps.

Over five years, the integration gradually proceeded. As
time went by, there was less "gapping" or "blanking out"; and

when she did gap, Cathy learned how to stay as present as possible while other personalities emerged. Eventually, she was even occasionally able to explore the gapping periods without therapeutic intervention and retain some memory.

## EPILOGUE

Cathy has learned to use her back pain as an indicator of her mental health. Before her back gets really painful, there are often several days of increasing tension; or, conversely, a particularly stressful event may precipitate the pain acutely. At that point, very often all she needs is minimal stimulation with acupuncture.

In a typical session of this kind she will start to shake and cry almost immediately then, after a minute or two — her words beginning to slur a bit — she will let us know that she is at the threshold. At that point, we need do no more than encourage her to try to stay present, and let anyone else come through who wants to. We may talk to one or two different personas — usually Grist will be one of them — and after ten or fifteen minutes, there is a recognizable shift and Cathy's whole body relaxes. Then she'll go off to sleep and generally awakes pain-free.

It seems clear in retrospect that Cathy's pain, like Donna's, signalled — and still signals — the need for other parts of herself to have expression. After this kind of session, the change in her demeanour is quite dramatic. Gone is the chronic pain and the pained appearance and behaviour; in its place is a lively, happier woman. As of this writing, Cathy is functioning well, is off all medications, and has full movement in her previously stiff neck.

Cathy's case was extraordinary, yet in fact her pain was no different from anyone else's. In every case, chronic pain points to a deeper reality which wants to emerge into consciousness. It is a call for a transformation of the small self to a larger self. For those who take the time to explore it, pain can become the mystical fire which transforms and gives meaning to life.

Chapter 26

# SYNCHRONICITY

*Acausal interconnectedness is to psychology
what quantum reality is to physics. Phenomena
occur not on the basis of cause and effect,
but on the basis of meaning.*

— Stephan Hoeller

*I*f, as science suggests, the universe is an infinitely cor-
related system, then every event is in some way related to every
other event. As conscious beings, we have the ability to recognize
those connections, and to ascribe meaning to the relationships
between events. Carl Jung, one of the founders of psychoanalysis,
coined the term synchronicity to describe the experience — which
many people are familiar with — of intuiting a connection between events which might otherwise be seen as mere coincidence.

Jung suggested that a sense of "meaning" arises when an
outer event occurs in such a way that it coincides with an inner
event — or inner archetypal image — and that choosing to take
a perspective which results in a continued sense of meaning, can
become a fundamental guiding principle for our lives. This idea
is not new of course, and has been echoed by others, but it can
extraordinarily difficult to find a sense of meaning when events
are destructive or horrific. One man who found such a way was
Victor Frankl, a psychiatrist who survived the Nazi concentration camps, and whose understanding of healing comes from
direct experience. He concluded that a man's attitude toward
suffering had a lot to do with his survival, and that finding
meaning in bad experiences was the key to spiritual healing. In
"Man's Search for Meaning" Dr. Frankl coined the term "lo-

gotherapy" to refer to the reframing process which gives rise to the sense of meaning, and founded a whole new school of psychiatry based on the idea.

If Frankl's experiences could stimulate us to look for connections and meaning in more mundane events, we might be astonished at the results. Of course, in order to make such connections, we have to be willing to "look with new eyes," and pay attention to those otherwise meaningless coincidences which occur from time to time. The effort to shift perspective allows us to do away with the inoperative notion of "cause and effect" in multifaceted problems such as chronic illness.

In many ways, healing involves just this shift from meaninglessness to meaning — from "coincidence" to "synchronicity." To begin with, our symptoms appear to have no meaning but as we explore them, we begin to make connections between our inner reality and the manifestations of our illness. Sometimes the connections can be so complex and profound that they go far beyond ourselves.

In the story which follows, the synchronous connections seemed to impact more on me than on Fred — the individual in question — and as the story unfolded I could do little more than shake my head in awe at the wonder and complexity of the universe. By the time I put it all together, I realized there were no more pigeonholes into which I could put the whole experience.

FRED : MULTIPLE INJURIES

Fred was a fifty-year-old trucker with thirty years of long-distance trucking behind him, and he had loved every minute of it. He was easy-going, solid, down-to-earth and utterly lacking in airs. His distinctive vocabulary and speech had been finely honed in various roadside cafes and bars. Fred first caught my attention because he sat back and out of the way, perhaps out of shyness, as though he just didn't want to be seen. His efforts to be absent seemed to make him all the more present.

Fred had been badly injured in a head-on collision one night in midwinter on the highway outside of Winnipeg. It was a bitterly cold prairie night and the road was icy. The last thing he recalled was seeing headlights coming at him, and then blackness.

When he came around he found himself sitting in the cab of his truck, wondering what had happened. When he tried to move, he couldn't. His right foot was jammed at an unnatural angle under the brake pedal; his left knee was smashed against the steering column; and his sternum had been crushed into the wheel. Worst of all, moving his left hip even a fraction caused him the most intense pain, pain which radiated right up his back and down his leg.

Still, it was a moment or two before he understood what had happened. When it registered that he had been in a major crash and was badly hurt, a few minutes of cautious experiment revealed he was also immobilized. There was little he could do but wait and hope: he couldn't move and it was twenty-five degrees below zero outside. Finally, after what seemed an eternity, rescue and ambulance crews, alerted by a passing driver, arrived and cut him out of the truck.

Fred had several injuries, including a lacerated liver, a broken right femur, a crushed right ankle, a fractured left hip, and a crushed vertebra. His back, left hip and right leg were operated on at once and he spent the next few weeks in hospital. Then after leaving acute care he faced months of physiotherapy, hydrotherapy, and physical rehabilitation.

It was about four years after his accident that Fred was referred to us. He still suffered from pain in his back, left hip, right leg and ankle, and had great difficulty bearing any weight on his right leg. He was taking anti-inflammatories, pain killers, muscle relaxants and an antidepressant — none of which he thought were doing him much good. In fact, he said he found himself increasingly debilitated and despondent.

The whole experience seemed to have altogether beaten him somehow, and despite intense physical rehabilitation, he was unable to get going again. More debilitating still, he faced an overwhelming anxiety which prevented him from getting into the cab of a truck. Since driving was Fred's only interest, his fear was all the more alarming to him and left him with no hope or sense of direction for the future.

When we first met, I talked to Fred at some length about the last moments he could recall before the collision and was struck by a peculiar detail which he mentioned quite casually. He said that right after the impact, while he was sitting dazed in the cab, just before he passed out, he had turned his head to the left and noticed someone looking in the side window. The man was a total stranger, fairly old — around seventy, he thought — with long greying hair, a lined and weathered face and deeply tanned skin; possibly Native, he added, nonchalantly. The man didn't say or do anything, just looked in the window and then moved off, as mysteriously as he'd appeared.

Now what, I thought, was an old man doing out on the highway in sub-zero weather at night, wordlessly looking into the windows of crashed trucks? Did he just happen to be passing by? Was he the one who called for help? Or was he a figment of Fred's imagination?

There was no way of knowing, but I filed the information away for future reference. Then I took a little closer look at Fred, and noticed that he too could be First Nations. My curiosity was piqued by the peculiar story he had related, and particularly by the calm, almost disinterested manner in which he had told it. It was all a little odd. I decided to take the bold approach.

"Is there any First Nations in your background, Fred?" I asked as casually as I could.

"Why do you want to know?" he countered suspiciously.

"It's nothing really," I assured him, "just that the man looking in the window seemed to be Native, and I just wondered if you were too." I tried to imply it was really not important.

"Well my mother once told me my dad was Sioux, but I don't really know ... I never met him. ... He wasn't ever around." Fred seemed embarrassed. I did not press the point further, trusting that a thorough exploration of the void might sort things out. But I made a mental note. If Fred had a Sioux background, he certainly wasn't advertising it. Not that that was so surprising: it's common enough for people to lose touch with their roots in our heterogenous culture, and he'd never really known his father. Still, I was interested by the suggestion that perhaps Fred had taken on a persona which did not represent his totality.

For the first while, Fred seemed quite suspicious of us, preferring to sit back and observe. When he finally did begin to work, though, he seemed committed to it: he breathed deeply to enter the void and stayed calm as the familiar shaking began. Soon it became apparent that he was not entirely present. He seemed to have gone off somewhere: his eyes flicked back and forth as if he were dreaming and he became less accessible, as if his initial physical withdrawal from the process was now being repeated psychically. After a few moments we lost contact completely as he headed off into the hidden recesses of the void.

Something significant seemed to be happening, however, so I didn't want to interfere, trusting that Fred would be able to recall what was going on when he came back. I waited for a few minutes after his return before broaching the subject but found that he could remember nothing. Nor did he seem to be particularly interested. After such a compelling experience, here again was that strange nonchalance. Something must have gone on though because before we started the next session, Fred admitted being frightened of returning to the void.

"Are we going to do the same thing as last time?" he asked.

"Why? Do you have a problem with it?" I returned his question.

"Well, I'm not sure I want to do it again."

"Why?" I asked. "What are you afraid of?"

"I don't know," he said. "I can't explain it." Fred's confession of fear was in direct contrast to his seeming nonchalance and posed a dilemma. If he was so easy-going, then why the fear? And if he was scared, why did he appear so placid? Something didn't add up.

In spite of his reservations, Fred eventually summoned the courage to return to the void several times during his stay with us, each time achieving an altered state of consciousness without being able to recall much about it afterwards. Acupuncture combined with a few minutes of deep breathing allowed him a gradual entry into the void. When he arrived, his eyes would flicker and he'd begin to shift his body from side to side, back and forth, and his breathing would become heavy and laboured. And later, all he claimed to remember about these episodes was that just *before* entering the void, he felt he was back in the cab of his truck, saw headlights approaching, then sensed someone was looking in his window. Then everything went black.

Fred's post-void disorientation always lasted several minutes, and although we could converse with him intelligently during that time, he would often not recall these conversations later. While in this state, he seemed to be present and rational, although later he would forget what had transpired. His memory seemed to drop from him from moment to moment as we spoke, much like a dream might evaporate upon awakening.

## THE GREY STONE

A few days after Fred arrived, I was walking across the parking lot, and a small heart-shaped grey stone caught my eye. As I bent to look at it more closely, it occurred to me that it was just the sort of stone that my wife, Cherie, would enjoy. She has always loved stones, particularly ones which have interesting shapes, colours, or markings; and since Cherie was with us at the clinic that day, I decided to pick it up and give it to her. I put the stone in my pocket and walked inside to find her sitting at the dining room table. When I gave her the stone, she looked totally shocked and put her hand over her heart as if to indicate the event had great meaning.

"What's the matter?" I asked, looking at her in astonishment.

"You won't believe this, Michael," she said, "but I've just been with Fred, and the most extraordinary thing happened."

"What's the stone got to do with it?" I persisted. "I just thought you would like it. See? It's shaped like a heart."

"Well, listen," said Cherie. "I was talking to Fred about his experiences here when he said something which literally blew me away".

"Well, carry on," I said, feeling my spine begin to tingle with a rising charge of excitement.

"Well, Fred seemed a bit spacey but no more than usual. He was sitting across from me looking perfectly Fred-like, if you know what I mean, when suddenly his eyes changed. They took on a deeper — how can I describe it? — a more profound expression. He looked me right in the eye and his voice went deeper — like he was a different person — then he said, 'My name is Greystone. I am an elder of my people. I saw the Raven you carry when I first got here — at the first night's meeting.'"

Cherie was electrified. For years she had carried the image of a Raven in her mind's eye as a power symbol but had no idea that the image might be real and even visible to others. The image of a raven was definitely significant to her but it wasn't something she talked about or acknowledged to many people. It certainly wasn't something she would usually have discussed with a relative stranger.

'Greystone' had continued: "I have a message for you. It is time for you to re-connect with your people. Soon you should go to where Raven lives and put your bare feet on the earth."

"You see?" said Cherie. "I get a message from a person called 'Greystone' — who is Fred but really isn't Fred, if you know what I mean — about the raven I carry which he says he sees, then you walk in here out of the blue and give me a grey stone shaped like a heart. What am I supposed to think?"

"I don't know," I said. "But I sure would be interested in what Fred has to say about it."

The next time Fred came to the acupuncture room he seemed entirely his usual self. I wanted to broach the subject of the grey stone, but wasn't quite sure how to begin. Since he hadn't mentioned anything to me about Greystone, I knew it might not be appropriate for me to raise the subject. If he was conscious of Greystone, he was obviously not in the habit of sharing him; and if he wasn't conscious of him, he might think I was crazy. I decided to try an open-ended question.

"Tell me, Fred" I said, "is there anything else you want to say or that you can recall about the person who looked into the truck just after the accident."

"No, there isn't," Fred replied. "I have no idea who he was or why he was there."

"Do you think he might be someone you know?" I asked cryptically. "I mean, there you were, badly injured, and it's twenty-five below zero. Who would be out there in that kind of weather, and then disappear? It's mysterious isn't it?"

"I really don't know what you mean," Fred said, in a way that implied he knew all-too-well what I meant. I decided to drop the subject and back off.

## HIDDEN POTENTIAL

Fred left us with his pain level down several notches. From a purely physical point of view, his improvement was greater than anyone had expected. I had the feeling however, that Fred's real work had only just begun. Because of the serious injury to his right ankle, it still seemed very unlikely that he would regain his former level of physical ability. He still had great difficulty weight-bearing on that leg, and was forced to use a cane to negotiate daily life. There was no way he could seriously contemplate returning to truck driving, so he would have to find another focus and occupation in his life.

Greystone seemed the obvious thing to explore. I had the distinct sense that Fred knew all about Greystone but did not want to acknowledge him. Perhaps it was a mark of his respect for his alter ego; or perhaps he was afraid of being shunned by a culture which has difficulty accepting such things. Whatever the reason, his shyness seemed a metaphor for the greater hiddenness of his life: to not be seen for who he really was. Since Fred never returned to the clinic, we never got the chance to work with him again. Was he conscious of this alter ego, or was he not? We probably will never know, because the one who knew chose not to talk about it. Yet the question hung in my mind.

## BAREFOOT IN THE PARK

Two weeks after Fred left us, Cherie and I went for a day hike in the hills around Victoria. We spent the day walking in the forest, and climbing until we reached rocky out-croppings and alpine meadows. Up there, the view of the Olympic Mountains to the south was breathtaking. To the west, some dark heavy clouds swept toward us threatening a seriously wet, windy evening but, for the time being, sun and showers, light and dark, mingled.

We sat down to drink in the view and rest for a few minutes before beginning the walk back home, and without any prompting, we both took off our shoes and socks and put our feet into the thick mossy carpet covering the ground. As we sat there, the big clouds gradually closed in, obscuring the view and bringing the temperature down sharply. Shivering in the sudden coolness, my immediate impulse was to get up and move before the weather really closed in.

But something seemed to hold us captive in that place as if suspended in time, waiting for some magic to happen. Then something did happen. For a brief moment, the black clouds separated, a stream of sunlight broke through the darkness and a familiar call broke the silence. Through the break in the clouds appeared two large and magnificent ravens.

We were spellbound. We sat there transfixed on the ground watching as these incredible creatures circled down and landed on the ground not twenty feet from us. They both looked directly at us for a moment, then, as quickly as they came, they were gone, off into the wind and the clouds. I looked over to Cherie and she looked back at me and to our surprise, we both found ourselves crying. Ten minutes later the clouds which had seemed so menacing completely cleared away, leaving a calm sunny evening for our homeward walk. We heard the ravens in the distance as we walked along, calling to us. To me, it seemed like a reminder to stay conscious. The threatened rains never came.

# AFTERWORD

## Thoughts about diagnosis and treatment

This book is a review of some of my experiences with clients over the past ten years. Those experiences have led me to conclusions which, by any conventional medical yardstick, are nothing short of heresy. Yet they are real enough, and speak to an understanding which is becoming increasingly important to those in search of healing. The experience of working with people in the void has been so profound that I feel it has transformed my consciousness. In the process, many of the sacrosanct tenets of my professional training in medicine have fallen by the wayside.

For example, I now question the value of intervention and no longer believe that diagnosis, as such, has much value in chronic illness. Diagnosis labels people as "not-normal" in some way, and denies the validity and immediacy of their experience. If I say you have "arthritis," I take away the immediacy of your experience of pain, and present you instead with a fairly meaningless generalization. If I say you have "dissociative disorder," the word disorder implies there is something wrong, and that "normal" people don't dissociate. In sum, it seems to me that in chronic illness at least, diagnosis is generally unhelpful and disempowering.

Nor do I any longer believe in the magic bullet. I was trained in a model of single diagnosis and the treatment of symptoms, which I now know misses the point. Anything we put in our mouths with the aim of eradicating symptoms misses the point. It matters not whether it is a drug, a herb, or a homeopathic remedy. Our intention is all that is important. If the intention is to eradicate symptoms, symptoms may be eradicated, but in the long run, healing may be deferred.

I no longer believe in listening to endless stories of victimization. Somewhere along the line, we become the architects of our experience, and by loitering in our own story we perpetuate any illness we might have. Talking is fine for a while, and everyone needs to have their story heard by a sympathetic ear, but there comes a time we must get into the body if we want to heal the body. When health providers try to be better listeners, they often end up being endless listeners: nothing new occurs, nothing changes. Eventually people forget that in order to live they must move on, and so symptoms become entrenched. Rather than talking endlessly, it might be better to observe the symptoms without judgement, remain in the immediacy of the moment, and allow the experience to teach us.

The extraordinary experiences in the void suggest to me that in fact there is no stasis, only repression, that everyone has unknown hidden potential waiting to be found, and that the doorway to discovery is contained in life's more painful experiences. To go in and discover what the self has to offer is the biggest gift we can give ourselves. Such a journey can give meaning to our lives beyond our wildest imagination.

# Appendix

# POEMS

# DIVINUM EST OPUS SEDARE DOLOREM
# (CONVERSATIONS ON PAIN: II)

*David Bosomworth*

## I.

*Pain*, restless for a host, darkened my doorstep,
   passed o'er my threshold, so crudely carved
     for welcoming visitants from my history,
       like *Pleasure, Anger, Joy* and *Fear*.

All invitees were there, the evening table spread
   by boarders, *Mind, Body,* and *Spirit,* three
     settlers in my Self's fine home,
       who lent me constant company
         providing cheer.

They knew not I had ranked them in myself as friends,
   yet meant that different tasks done for me,
     for selfish ends, you might well say;
       yet they were thus so priorized,
         but loved the same.

So at this rugged threshold they did promptly stand,
   When suddenly this *Pain* emerged from darkness,
     bringing *Chaos* to my fine estate,
       along with *Mystery,* through
         my iron garden gate.

In rude and mattered-moment, *Charity* went out the door,
   and honoured *Hope,* feeling some helpless hollowness
     took *Trust* and *Faith* up to the fire-escape;
       and *Pleasure* simply disappeared,
         spilling giggles to the air.

And I was left with just a minor motley-crew of few
   whom I'd invited, just to give this night
     in life a simmer and some spice;
       *Anger, Fear,* and *Arrogance*
         with *Loneliness* remained.

There were others too, but mostly of the "tarnished" kind,
so I was on my own, uncertain of my future fate,
for *Pain* and never visited my *Self* before,
nor had it ever approached
my welcoming door.

So I forthwith appealed to *Mind, Body, Spirit,* helpers-three,
in this bizarre development, to quickly assist me;
but they had changed, reframed themselves,
and *Me, Myself* and *I* became a weight
of Self-imposed disharmony.

My *Mind* unleashed an unfamiliar sense of paranoia, persecution,
at its best, while boldly *Body* bent cruelly played
a victim role, in spite of former endless praise;
and *Spirit* soon refused to Be; a "rescuer,"
invited *Pain* to stay.


## II.

So I was forced to face what Pain produced within my Home.
and this, the terrible triad of tremendous power
to rescue, victimize, then persecute,
was not my habit, not my style.
My house was not my Home.

For *Happiness* had been moved, beyond my gate, to tears,
And *Confidence* came forth as *Cowardice*;
*Meaningfulness* had viewed the Void;
treasured guests, through *Pain*
were, all around, reframed.

Then for one small moment, *breathing paused; sleepers awakened;*
*Yearning* yawned; action froze and darkness moved;
and *Pain* reached out its withered hand
to touch my heart with saddened grace,
... and I saw *Wisdom* in its face.

A "Presence" moved around my rooms, around my house, my home;
I heard the song of meadow-lark, sad cries of spirits
in the dark; not here, but there, beyond my rooms;
indeed, beyond this phantom, *Pain*;
beyond the Moon.

# III.

Just what I felt, I cannot say; too few the words for *Mystery*,
but now I know that *Pain* arrived with words from *Wisdom* deep
to share a simple meal with my self-history;
I felt, in time, its perilous power
graciously subdue.

So I listened for the sighing of a breeze
and felt the coolness of refreshing dew.
*Pain* had come to me, not to rob my soul, not to ravage all
I held as true, but to open my eyes
to that which lay beyond my Self,
my House, my meanings
and my truths;

to sharpen my awareness of the paradox of Life;
the Sun which carves a shadowed day.
the Moon's reflected night light;
and to search for understanding,
when *Pain* was first in sight,
why my guests ran out
in horror to the
blindness of
the night;

to muse upon a certainty; one I won't forget:
that I may see sought *Wisdom* through
a touch of some regret.
These are lessons
tried and true,
set in print
for me and
you.

# FEAR

*Holly Ladouceur*

It is dark in here,
I do not understand.
The cloud is closing in,
My life is at hand.
It is cold in here,
I shiver where I stand.
The pain is squeezing me,
I feel that I am damned.
It is scary in here,
And I cannot command.
The fear inside of me,
Has gotten out of hand.

My Mind has deceived me,
Led me far away.

Buried all the memories,
to haunt me to this day.

The world has shut off,
Feelings put aside.
Emotions left unknown,
In this way that I could hide.

Round and round the world went,
'Til the wall came crashing down.

Memories came flooding in,
So frightening did they seem.
But now the sunshine up above,
Can give me just a beam.

Open up my broken heart,
Sew up all the seams.
Let me be the person,
That I've always dreamed.

# TRANSFORMATION

*Holly Ladouceur*

I had a business doing well
Got very sick three long years ago
Started by the car accident,
And the medicine for control,
My body hurt and my mind in pain,
My being began to dwindle.
I lost my body, heart and soul,
wishing for life to rekindle.

The pain that grew inside of me,
Took me to the edge.
Everything the doctors did,
Put in a bigger wedge.
They cut me open, took me apart,
And left me for the dead.

As I grew worse day by day,
My home became my bed. I lost it
all, my work, my goals,
My dreams and visions quest.
I faced the darkest side of life,
Where fears and shadows rest.
Until the day came,
I finally realized,
This is my life, my heart, my soul,
That has been paralyzed.

Take control and don't let go,
Keep the urge to fight.
Wait on the will of Heaven
Then spread your wings for flight.

# PAIN

*Norma D.*

To describe my pain and what it does to me would be impossible to do
It keeps me company through thick and thin, through daylight & starlight
It has the ability to slow time especially at night
It can hold your breath or speed it up
It can throw you to the ground or crumple you like a dead leaf
Pain can bend and warp your thoughts
Telling you that you would be better off
By yourself or maybe that you should not live
It can make you buy pills you didn't mean to
It calls to you constantly and unrelentingly
Never giving in always winning
Pain can pull you from society
It softens your muscles and your will
It confuses you, makes you mad, makes you cry
It makes you want to die: but no that must be a lie
Because you would be insane to want to die
But then again I might be insane.....


# DAY IN DAY OUT

*Norma D.*

Day in day out
It covers me like a thick dark cloud
Tumbling about me
But never getting thinner sometimes thicker
But never ending
Making attempts to end the pain
With a soup of drugs only stirs the cloud,
As impossible to push away
As it would be
To remove a thunder cloud with your breath.
Dreams of lifting the cloud
Close at hand
But always out of reach.

# A MONSTER

*Norma D.*

The faceless monster deep inside my mind
Brought to life by the fear of future time
This deep terror runs black and cold
For what will this monster do, it is so old

A vision that comes toward my eye
Of nothingness deep as the sea as large as the sky
How can this be the terror I feel
It cannot be touched but is very real

If only the courage and strength could be found
To stand up to what will come around
Try not to cry, try real hard not to cower
Deflate all the negativity of this great power
Learn to face each monster present and past
With bravery and guts that will last

Oh to be wise beyond all time
to face the monster with peace of mind
as each day comes and each day goes
The sickness of fear takes its toll
Finding power within to fight this guy
Weakens and tires and flattens, but why?

The question of why is asked with fear in my face
Why won't the monster shrink and give me some space
Did in some past life I commit a grave sin
That now I am punished by monsters within

The more desperate I search for an answer it seems
The further away from a truth I am pulled
My monster that is strong and scary old and wise
Knows the truth of my eventual demise

The secret he holds won't be clear until the end
For the monster is selfish and childish and not a friend
If I ever give in to this powerful force
The inevitable death of self will take its course

This monster requires my death to be free
The door to this creature is deep inside of me
Has the lock of life to keep it shut tight
One day the monstrous creature will win the fight

The lock that life has on this door to hell
Will be picked loose by the demons of present and past
And death will finally release my fear at last
This dark and sad creature will then go with my pain

## LIVING BUT NOT ALIVE

*Norma D.*

Living but not alive
dead but not dead
Breathing only to feed the pain
Going forward only to end at the beginning

Feeling obsessed with death but have no focus
afraid to live through the torment
Tormented with the lack of life
A profound blindness for any future

Trying to do what others expect
With no idea of what to expect of myself
Burning with resentment and anger of now
Being stuck in today because tomorrow is today again.

## DESPAIR

Despair is a long black tunnel
That sucks life from you
smothering
With its heaviness like thick tar
Knowing that despair is at hand
makes
Little difference to how it feels
No one can truly know the
pure darkness

Of despair unless it has been experienced
Words seem inadequate for such a devastating feeling
How easy
It would be to give in
And let despair win for it is
Strong

Maybe stronger than me, maybe not
I guess I will know
When
I am either dead or alive
For those
Are the only two outcomes from this
Blackness


# THE VOID

*Norma D.*

I am on the edge
Of a void
Deep, dark, silent
No life within

It would only take one slip
Then I would tumble
For all eternity
Unable to stop
Or
To grasp a hold of anything
On and on
With no end in sight

*Please note: The preceding poems were written by individuals who have braved the void and felt moved to write about their experience. Although they have kindly agreed to allow me to print their writings, their specific journeys do not appear anywhere in the book.*

"Abused Boys Suffer More Sequelae than Girls." Interview with Dr. J. Turner. In *Canadian Family Practice*, Feb. 7, 1994.

Bolen, Jean Shinolda. *Crossing to Avalon; a woman's midlife pilgrimage*. Scarborough: Harper Collins, 1995.

Castaneda, Carlos. *A Separate Reality*. New York: Simon & Schuster, 1971.

Finkell, K.C. "Sex Abuse and Incest." *Canadian Family Physician*, vol . 40, May 1994.

Flaws, Bob. "Sex Abuse and TCM." *Journal of Chinese Medicine*, no. 42, May 1993.

Frankl, Victor E. *Man's Search for Meaning; an introduction to logotherapy*. New York, Simon & Schuster, 1959.

Grimm, Jakob and Wilhelm. *Grimm's Fairy Tales*. New York: M.A. Donohue & Co., 1920.

Harner, Michael James. *The Way of the Shaman: a guide to power and healing*. New York: Bantam Books, 1982.

Harper, Tom. *The Uncommon Touch: an investigation of spiritual healing*. Toronto: McClelland and Stewart, 1995.

Hoeller, Stephan A. "Exorcism, Inner and Outer." *Critique: A Journal Questioning Consensus Reality*.

Hubbard, Robert. *Dianetics*. Los Angeles: Bridge Publishers, 1992.

Jarrett, Lonny S. "Constitutional Type and the Internal Tradition of Chinese Medicine." *American Journal of Acupuncture:* vol.21, no.1, 1993.

Kluft, Richard P. "An Update on Multiple Personality Disorder." *Hospital and Community Psychiatry,* vol.38, no.4 (April 1987).

Lewis, C.S. *The Magician's Nephew*. New York: Macmillan, 1988, 1955.

Monroe, Robert. *Journeys out of the Body*. New York: Doubleday, 1971.

Mood, John J.L. *Rilke on Love and other Difficulties: translations and considerations of Rainer Maria Rilke*. New York: W.W Norton & Co., 1975.

Moody, Raymond A. *Life after Life: the investigation of a phenomenon*. Boston: G.K. Hall, 1977.

Phillips, J.B. *The Gospels*. Trans. J.B. Phillips. Frome and London: Butler & Tanner Ltd., for Geoffrey Bless Ltd. 1952. 1956 edition.

Sheldrake, Rupert. *A New Science of Life: the hypothesis of formative causation*. London: Paladin Grafton Books, 1985.

Smith, Margaret. *Ritual Abuse: what it is, why it happens, how to help*. New York: Harper Collins, 1993.

Stein, Robert. *Incest and Human Love: the betrayal of the soul in psychotherapy*. Dallas: Spring Publishers, 1984.

Ziegler, Alfred J. "Illness as descent into the body." In *Meeting the Shadow*, Connie Zweig and Jeremiah Abrams, eds. Los Angeles: Jeremy P. Tarcher, Inc., 1991.

# Index

## A

## B